## Praise for *Helping Patients Outsmart Overeating*

"Despite evidence that diets don't work for sustaining weight loss, many doctors are unaware of other options for their 'overweight' patients. This book provides more effective ways to end dysfunctional eating and promote healthy attitudes and behaviors around food. Using these insights and strategies from the field of eating disorders treatment, medical professionals can more successfully help patients who are challenged by overeating."

—**Leigh Cohn**, M.A.T., C.E.D.S., editor-in-chief,
*Eating Disorders: The Journal of Treatment and Prevention*

"Finally, a weight-inclusive book aimed at physicians and health care providers that puts the focus on health, rather than weight. All too often patients avoid seeing their doctors because of self-shame around their weight, which in the long run hurts health. This compassionately written book describes the psychological complexity around dysregulated eating, weight bias, and self-care. Ultimately, health care providers will learn how they can help their patients, with the bonus that they may discover solutions to their own unresolved issues around weight and eating. And who better to learn this from than one of their own—written by a therapist, Karen R. Koenig, and a physician, Paige O'Mahoney?"

—**Evelyn Tribole**, M.S., R.D., coauthor of *Intuitive Eating*

"At a time when physicians are challenged with less time in the exam room, and more patients struggling with unhealthy diets, this book may be the psychological tool that finally helps motivate healthy change. If your doctor doesn't have this book, bring it to your next appointment."

—**Heidi Godman**, health journalist, host of
*Health Check with Heidi Godman*

"This wise and insightful book is an invaluable resource for a wide range of professionals who treat seemingly intractable weight and eating problems. As a clinician and researcher of the diet-binge cycle for many decades, I welcome both its clarity and its compassion in guiding patients to a healthier relationship with food and their bodies."

—**Emily Fox-Kales**, Ph.D., author, *Body Shots: Hollywood
and the Culture of Eating Disorders*; founder and director,
Feeding Ourselves

"A handy resource for all health care practitioners who want to help patients address their eating in a compassionate, sensitive, and motivating way! This beneficial guide is filled with solid tips for facilitating a healthy mindset around food and weight and to-the-point chapter summaries from two health care providers who express their passion about quality care!"

—**Susan Albers**, M.D., clinical psychologist and
*New York Times* bestselling author of *EatQ* and
*Eating Mindfully*

# Helping Patients Outsmart Overeating

## Psychological Strategies for Doctors and Health Care Providers

KAREN R. KOENIG, M.ED., LCSW,
AND PAIGE O'MAHONEY, M.D., CHWC

ROWMAN & LITTLEFIELD
*Lanham • Boulder • New York • London*

Published by Rowman & Littlefield
A wholly owned subsidary of The Rowman & Littlefield Publishing Group, Inc.
4501 Forbes Boulevard, Suite 200, Lanham, Maryland 20706
www.rowman.com

Unit A, Whitacre Mews, 26-34 Stannary Street, London SE11 4AB

DISCLAIMER
While we hope that the information contained herein will be helpful to you, please note that this book is intended for informational and educational purposes only. For health care providers, the information may not be applicable or appropriate for every patient or practice situation. The authors do not provide medical or psychological assessment, advice, or individualized therapeutic interventions. This book is not intended to substitute for a health care provider's professional evaluation and assessment of an individual patient. Further, it is not intended to substitute for personal consultation with your health care provider regarding your individual medical or mental health situation. The authors and publisher specifically disclaim any and all liability arising directly or indirectly from the use of any information contained in this book. Mention of products, techniques, methods, resources, approaches, or other entities in this book does not indicate endorsement by the authors or publisher.

British Library Cataloguing in Publication Information Available

**Library of Congress Cataloging-in-Publication Data**
Names: Koenig, Karen R., 1947– author. | O'Mahoney, Paige, author.
Title: Helping patients outsmart overeating : psychological strategies for
    doctors and health care providers / Karen R. Koenig and Paige O'Mahoney.
Description: Lanham : Rowman & Littlefield, [2017] | Includes bibliographical
    references and index.
Identifiers: LCCN 2016025052 (print) | LCCN 2016026341 (ebook) |
    ISBN 9781442266629 (cloth : alk. paper) | ISBN 9781442266636 (electronic)
Subjects: LCSH: Eating disorders—Psychological aspects. |
    Food—Psychological aspects. | Physician and patient—Popular works |
    Medical personnel and patient—Popular works.
Classification: LCC RC552.E18 K633 2017 (print) | LCC RC552.E18 (ebook) |
    DDC 616.85/26—dc23
LC record available at https://lccn.loc.gov/2016025052

♾️™ The paper used in this publication meets the minimum requirements of American National Standard for Information Sciences—Permanence of Paper for Printed Library Materials, ANSI/NISO Z39.48-1992.

Printed in the United States of America

KRK: This book is dedicated in memoriam to my cousin, Laurie Dunn.

POM: To my family, former patients, clients, mentors, and teachers, who have inspired and nurtured this book.

# Contents

# Acknowledgments

Kudos to our agent, Janice M. Pieroni of Story Arts Management, who was behind the mission of this book 100 percent from the get-go. We thank Rowman & Littlefield and Suzanne Staszak-Silva for partnering with us to bring this book to fruition. Thanks as well to Grier Ferguson for administrative support, especially for her attention to detail, and to Tracy Tylka, Ph.D., for sharing her expertise on the research in this area.

Finally, we would like to thank the health and mental health professionals, researchers, patient advocates and others whose work we have highlighted throughout the pages of this book. We are grateful to them for helping to change the patient-provider conversation that traditionally has been about diets and weight, to one increasingly focused on promoting sustainable health and wellness through enhancement of patients' self-worth, self-compassion, self-efficacy and self-care no matter what their size.

# Foreword

As a lifestyle medicine practitioner, trained as both a physician and a health coach, I work with patients who want to lose weight and I teach physicians and health care providers how to work with patients on adopting regular exercise, nutritious eating patterns, and stress resiliency. I am acutely aware of the need for practical tools in this area. Paige and Karen have mapped out a play-by-play instruction manual on how to engage patients in their own self-care, with a focus on adopting healthy habits.

Research and clinical experience demonstrate that when patients focus on sustaining healthful behaviors versus losing weight, they are happier and healthier. How to accomplish this is not currently part of the medical school curriculum. However, we are trying to change that. This book is one big step forward in the journey to transform medical care. Practitioners can fill the gap in their own medical training by reading this book and learning how to speak to patients so that they will listen and, more importantly, so that they will tell you what they really need in order to feel and be well.

This book is truly a gift to those suffering from weight cycling and dys-regulated eating as well as a gift to those who care for these patients. As health care providers who themselves have struggled with useless diets and negative self-talk, these two authors have crafted a playbook for providers to empower patients and provide them with the tools and skills they desperately need and want. With engaging chapters and practical tips included in each, the reader is left feeling more confident about working with patients who are uncomfortable with their weight and with their eating patterns. This book is bound to help providers and patients, and might well help the nation to cure the obesity epidemic that plagues us. Congratulations to Paige and Karen for putting together such an easy to read, information-packed, practical approach to helping patients live a healthy life without obsessing about their weight.

Elizabeth Pegg Frates, M.D.
Director of Wellness Programming
Stroke Institute for Research and Recovery
Spaulding Rehabilitation Hospital
Assistant Professor, Part Time
Harvard Medical School

April 4, 2016

# Preface

February 12, 2015, was one of those glorious, warm, sparkling February days in Florida that those of us who live in more northern climes dream about all winter long. Karen and I sat across from one another at a comfortable café, talking as though we had known each other for years. I had devoured her books while seeking to resolve my own issues with food and eating and found her style, expertise, and perspectives tremendously helpful. Hoping to learn more about her approach, I had e-mailed Karen about attending one of her workshops in Sarasota. When the workshop was rescheduled, and as I was going to be near Sarasota anyway, we decided to meet for lunch. As we ate and shared our eating histories and perspectives, the creative energy between us grew and grew—and eventually evolved into this book for health professionals: doctors, nurses, nurse practitioners, dietitians, therapists, coaches, trainers, and others to whom patients look for better eating and health advice.

As an M.D., after years of observing how physicians, health care providers, and even patients often approach weight-related challenges as a failure of patient willpower and/or lack of motivation, I became interested in learning about the "eating psychology" approach used by eating disorder therapists like Karen. Through my studies, I began to understand that how and what patients *think* about food, eating, weight, and their body image, rather than *what* they eat, is often a major determinant of their permanent success in improving their relationship with food. The psychology of eating viewpoint is that *weight* concerns often (although certainly not always) are derived from *eating* problems, including chronic dieting, and that attempts to treat "overweight" must start with a patient's *thoughts, feelings, and behaviors.*

I hope, both professionally and personally, that you enjoy and benefit from our collaborative effort to empower and inspire physicians and health care providers to help patients achieve lasting success in ending their struggles with food, weight, and body image.

Paige O'Mahoney, M.D., CHWC, March 17, 2016

After writing six books on eating, weight, and body image, I swore I had nothing else to say on the subject and was planning to return to fiction writing—until I had lunch with Paige. Her passion and compassion convinced me that it was time to give voice to the clients with high weights in my psychotherapy practice who grumbled about how much they hated going to doctors or other health professionals and, therefore, often avoided doing so.

Until that lunch with Paige, all I could do was to try my hardest to empower these patients by blogging on the subject and encouraging them to share their feelings with their practitioners and express their needs for health care infused with respect, compassion, and patience. Collaborating on this book offers them so much more than any therapy session or therapist ever could. It is a means to, as Paige would say, change the conversation between healers and those who need healing with food and their bodies. I believe I speak on behalf of people with high weights when I say that, even when it looks as if they don't care a whit about their health, they desperately want to mend their broken relationships with food and their bodies and get on with having a great life. With equal fervor, I hope that this book is viewed by doctors and health care providers as a means to become the healers they set out to be.

Karen R. Koenig, M.Ed., LCSW, March 17, 2016

# Introduction

The purpose of this book is to help doctors and health care professionals treat patients with eating and weight concerns more successfully. Our aim is to enhance the mental and physical health of patients by educating their providers about practical, hands-on strategies, techniques, and tools from the fields of eating and success psychologies. These are approaches that we doubt you learned in your professional training, but they can make all the difference in treating your patients and helping them have a positive relationship with food and their bodies. The psychological principles that we teach for guiding patients toward wellness are timeless and enduring, unlike ever-changing scientific theories on exactly how to eat and exercise.

Our hope is that people with eating and weight concerns will also read this book and take its message (if not the book itself!) about their desire to be treated with dignity and respect no matter what their size or eating problems to their health care providers. Our intent is to give them validation and courage to be candid with their clinicians about what is and what isn't helpful to them in the provider-patient relationship. Through honest conversation, our aim is to put providers and patients on the same page about what will help them become successful in reaching their mutual goals.

*Helping Patients Outsmart Overeating* will teach you and your patients how to best use your limited time together to address behaviors such as binge eating, emotional and compulsive eating, mindless eating, run-of-the-mill overeating, and chronic weight cycling. Rest assured, we're not trying to turn doctors into eating disorders' therapists, nor do we view using basic psychological approaches during a medical visit as a substitute for patients getting additional, targeted clinical help for their eating problems.

The "psychology of eating," a term with which both providers and patients may be unfamiliar, is the study of how, when, and why we eat. It is not about "what" to eat, and this is not a book about nutrition. In a way, it's about everything but food—understanding the effect that mood, ingrained beliefs, emotions, stress, appetite cues, self-talk, trauma, social support, self-care, unconscious intrapsychic conflicts, a balanced lifestyle, and life skills have on our relationship with it. The "psychology of eating" is focused on enhancing mental health, mindfulness, self-care, emotional regulation, and life skills, which will lead to improved attunement to appetite, more nutritious food choices and appropriate food portions, and the development of consistent exercise habits to promote ongoing good health. Think of it as creating lasting change from the inside out, unlike diets, which promote temporary change from the outside in, assuming that a thinner body will lead to increased happiness.

Thought leaders in the field of eating disorders have known for more than three decades that it is less the "what" of eating than the "why" and "how" that make all the difference in people developing a positive relationship with food. The "psychology of eating" is mindful of nutrition, but it is not focused on calories, carbohydrates, fat and sugar grams. Its ultimate goal is to teach patients how to develop a positive, "normal" relationship with food, which means:

- Feeling deserving enough and empowered to take good care of one's body, which includes developing and sustaining internal motivation for this essential task.
- Holding a belief system and engaging in positive self-talk, which are congruent with and generate positive health practices.
- Not dieting or thinking of food in "good" or "bad" moralistic terms.
- Making health and wellness one's focus, not a number on the scale.
- Developing appetite attunement regarding hunger, food choice, and satiety.
- Ending emotional and compulsive eating.
- Using food primarily for nourishment and occasionally for pleasure.
- Developing effective life skills to increase self-care and manage stress and distress without turning to food, promoting consistency which helps sustain positive behavioral change.

- Resolving underlying, mostly unconscious, internal conflicts, which can otherwise interfere with attaining and sustaining eating and fitness-related goals.

*Helping Patients Outsmart Overeating* seeks to transform patients from being dysregulated eaters (restricting food which leads to overeating which leads to restricting food, etc.) into "normal" eaters—people who eat (mostly) when they are hungry, make nutritious and satisfying food choices, eat with awareness and an eye toward enjoyment, and put down their knives and forks when they have had enough. Though deliberately not weight focused, "psychology of eating" strategies set the stage for patients to end dysfunctional food patterns and eat more nutritiously, which may result in weight loss and maintenance of a natural, comfortable weight.

In this book, we are addressing patients who have eating attitudes or engage in eating behaviors which prevent them from feeling empowered, comfortable, sane, and relaxed around food. When we refer to "doctors" or "clinicians," our aim is to include all health care providers—nurses, nurse practitioners, dietitians, diabetes educators, therapists, eating and life coaches, and others—who care for patients with eating or weight concerns.

Our ultimate goals are to change the conversation between patient and professional (and among professionals), to advance the state of the art in the treatment of eating and weight concerns, and to support providers in successfully encouraging patients to improve their attitudes and habits around food in order to eat both "normally" *and* healthfully. This approach employs helpful practices from motivational theory, eating psychology, and success psychology, in order to empower and support patients in making cognitive, emotional, and behavioral changes that promote long-term health. A sample of this collective wisdom encourages health care providers to help patients by:

1. Focusing on both mental and physical health improvement, leading to enhanced patient self-efficacy and sustainable wellness, rather than on weight loss, as the ultimate goal.
2. Using motivational interviewing, appreciative inquiry, and other success-promoting methods that help patients take responsibility for setting and reaching realistic health goals.
3. Using words, tone, and body language that are constructive, engaging, empathic, honest, compassionate, realistic, respectful, and, above all, non-judgmental about weight and size.

4. Avoiding weight shaming, stigmatization, and lecturing or preaching about what they should or shouldn't put into their mouths or how vigorously they should exercise, and instead empowering patients to operate from a mindset of self-acceptance, self-compassion, and an internal locus of control.

5. Recognizing that eating and health concerns are highly complex, biopsychosocial phenomena, involving genetics, environment, life history, self-talk, temperament, emotions, psychology, biochemistry, trauma, and much more.

6. Understanding that the inability to resolve eating and weight concerns is often rooted in (conscious or unconscious) internal conflicts regarding worthiness and deservedness of good mental and physical self-care, and that sustained health maintenance takes root only after these conflicts are resolved.

7. Reinforcing that small, incremental steps count; practice makes progress (not perfection); consistent, constructive thoughts and behaviors lead to success; and it is more beneficial to focus on what patients are doing right than on what they are doing wrong or have yet to do.

8. Recognizing how trauma, abuse, neglect, poverty, class, race, poor self-efficacy, life skill deficits, depression and anxiety disorders, among myriad factors, often underlie or exacerbate eating issues, and helping them access appropriate help or treatment for these issues.

9. Listening to them talk about their physical ailments without turning them into "weight problems" (along with medical staff insisting they get weighed, this is higher-weight patients' most common complaint about doctors and health care practitioners).

10. Recognizing how clinicians' own eating or weight struggles or biases may color their attitudes in addressing patients' food issues and get in the way of providing effective and caring treatment.

*Helping Patients Outsmart Overeating* is written by an experienced pediatrician and a seasoned eating disorders' clinician, both of whom have had their own mega-eating struggles. Both authors have experienced the misery of yo-yo dieting, sneak eating, binge eating, food deprivation, weights traveling up and down the scale, and relationships with food that could at best be called dysfunctional and, at worst, downright self-destructive.

One of our major goals is to eliminate the blame and shame felt by both parties when patients fail to follow their health care providers' nutritional and activity-related advice for the long term. Playing the blame game is a barrier to clear and open communication and what providers and patients most want: successful, sustained improvement in wellness-promoting attitudes and behaviors.

*Providers are not to blame.* They attended medical, nursing, or other professional schools and entered their respective fields to prevent and cure illness and improve and save lives, not to spend an inordinate amount of time nagging and badgering patients into making healthy lifestyle changes (most of which their patients already know they need to make). Like the rest of our culture, most clinicians have been hoodwinked into believing in the long-term efficacy of diet programs, pills, and surgery. And many have also bought into our culture's rampant fat phobia and prejudice. How could they not?

*Patients are not to blame either.* They, too, have been conned by the diet industry and our culture's obsession with thinness rather than wellness. Anyone who has ever dieted is intimately acquainted with why restrictive eating doesn't work for the long term due to pervasive feelings of deprivation, the exhaustion of unending self-control challenges, metabolic compensation and weight-loss plateaus, and inevitable rebound eating. This pattern produces a repetitive diet-restrict-binge, "yo-yoing" cycle that often leads to energy depletion, frustration, feelings of helplessness, plummeting self-esteem, and a sense of despair, in addition to deleterious physical and metabolic consequences. Until our patients confront the psychological roots of this revolving-door pattern and develop more effective life skills and appropriate mindsets, admonitions to eat less and move more will do little to help them.

A major challenge in writing this book has been finding an appropriate term to describe the patients we seek to help. The most commonly used terms for this population in the medical vernacular are "overweight," "obese," or "morbidly obese." Because these terms reflect a judgmental, weight-normative approach and, therefore, carry negative connotations, they did not fit the bill. It's obvious that no patient wants to be called "obese," and even the seemingly innocuous "overweight" is a judgment that being in excess of a particular number means patients are automatically unhealthy, which is patently untrue. Many other factors, aside from weight, contribute to good or poor health.

Several studies on how patients feel about the terminology used to describe their weight and size by medical providers tell us that, indeed, language matters to them a great deal. Themes from research include avoidance of return medical appointments if doctors used stigmatizing language[1] and the fact that some populations might consider being called "overweight" and "obese" an indication that they are "unmotivated, depressed and do not care about themselves."[2]

The same difficulty is found with the term "weight problem," in that research cited in Chapter 3, "How Diets Kill Motivation and Make People Fatter," tells us that how much people weigh is not a particularly effective tool in measuring overall health. It is not weight per se that is the problem, but rather dysfunctional eating, sedentary lifestyles, and inadequate self-care strategies, along with other factors such as genetics and biology, which are not under the patient's voluntary control.

Lest you think that we are simply being excessively politically correct by challenging the common usage of "overweight" and "weight problems," we assure you that our sole purpose is to do what is in the best interest of patients to become healthier, not adhering to some model of political correctness. As the saying goes, when you're a hammer, everything looks like a nail. Using terminology that makes weight *the* problem will not lead to effective, holistic treatment or to a satisfactory, sustainable resolution of patients' eating problems. If it did, there would be no need for this book.

Our conviction is that words spring from beliefs. If we believe that something is wrong with the patient because they are outside of certain weight norms, we are making a negative judgment about them. Why not call them what they are: high or higher weight, which is descriptive without making a judgment? By taking a more weight-inclusive approach, providers enable themselves to see the patient in context, rather than simply as a number on the scale. Research indicates that this weight-inclusive approach is better for both patient and provider.[3]

Chapter 1 validates doctors' frustrations about patients not heeding their advice to eat less and move more, and Chapter 2 provides the patients' perspective of struggling—and, more often than not, failing miserably—to permanently improve their eating and health and their unhappiness with how doctors treat them and their weight concerns.

Chapter 3 presents evidence for why diets don't work for the long term and actually can make people regain more weight than they originally lost—not to mention how dieting increases stress and frustration and lowers self-efficacy, which often triggers mindless eating. In Chapter 4 we describe common personality traits of the dysregulated eater, as well as the effects of abuse, trauma, and mood disorders that can exacerbate dysregulated eating behaviors, and in Chapter 5 we focus on how to help patients become "normal" and nutritious eaters.

Chapter 6 gets up close and personal, describing how practitioners' own battles with food and the scale may get in the way of discussing patients' similar concerns. Chapter 7 details how the doctor-patient collaboration can produce successful, lasting resolution of patients' eating and weight concerns through the use of appropriate, nonjudgmental language, empathy, compassion, and motivational interviewing, among other strategies. Finally, Chapter 8 discusses how collegial and ancillary support networks and learning about Intuitive Eating, the weight-inclusive approach to health, and Lifestyle Medicine principles can support both patients and clinicians in reaching their goals.

At the end of *Helping Patients Outsmart Overeating*, there is a bibliography and listing of helpful books, websites, and resources for patients and practitioners for ongoing education and support.

# 1

# Why Doctors Are Frustrated

## (Help, I'm Losing Patience with My Patients!)

- Description of doctors' and providers' chief complaints when working with patients who have eating and weight concerns
- What treatment approaches are not working with these patients
- Special challenges in working with pediatric patients
- Who, if anyone, is to blame for escalating weights
- A new direction for treatment of eating and weight concerns

As physicians and health care providers, we have devoted our lives to helping others. We have spent years in training, and more years staying abreast of the most recent developments in medicine to promote wellness and heal our patients. As a profession, we can cure many diseases that killed people a mere half century ago, we have incredible technologies that allow us to fix problems inside the human body in a minimally invasive way, and scientists have even mapped the human genome. Yet we feel powerless to help our patients achieve and maintain a natural, comfortable weight with our current nutritional and exercise recommendations, medications, and surgery. We confront that failure daily in our busy practices, operating rooms, and hospitals.

Our patients experience even greater frustration. Some have struggled all their lives to lose weight and not regain it. They feel fed up and beaten down by decades of dieting, battling the scale, and watching the number on it continue to creep up. Some have tried to diet but gave up when their weight plateaued and they stopped shedding pounds. Now they no longer even try to watch what they eat. Desperate or depressed, they enter medical offices complaining about aching knees, hips, and back, their high blood pressure medications not working as well as they'd hoped, what a struggle it is to lose and keep off even a few pounds, and how easy it is to put them back on.

To both our credit and our detriment, many providers take this scenario personally, as we worry about the consequences of our patients' lifestyle choices and health problems, both for them and for our ability to care for them. We are apprehensive that their self-care behaviors will compromise the best possible outcomes of any intervention, despite our dedication and best efforts. Worse, we suspect that this downward health spiral will only become more of a problem as our patients age. "Why," we ask ourselves and our colleagues repeatedly, "is this so hard, and why are our efforts not working?"

Let's look at a typical case that a primary care physician might encounter in order to examine and understand what's not working well in the relationship between patient and provider. Say Ms. Smith, a fifty-nine-year-old female executive, has been your patient for the past twenty-four years. She presents with a primary complaint of bilateral knee and hip pain, which has worsened progressively over the past two months and is exacerbated by climbing stairs and walking for long periods. This is interfering with her ability to move efficiently through airports as part of her busy travel schedule. Her medical history is significant for "pre-diabetes," hypertension, obstructive sleep apnea, and episodic depression and anxiety. She has gained 4 kg (almost 9 pounds) since her last wellness check twelve months ago. Today, her height is 5'3" and her weight is 85 kg, or 187 pounds. She is distressed by her weight gain, particularly because she suspects that the extra pounds are aggravating her knee and hip pain, not to mention her other health concerns.

Despite the fact that she has been on and off diets for the past thirty years and has lost a substantial number of pounds each time, she has regained it all, and her weight continues to rise as her energy level continues to wane. When you ask for more details about her efforts, Ms. Smith reports that her joint pain interferes with her ability to exercise comfortably, and she feels caught in a vicious cycle. She tells you that her sleep apnea prevents her from getting a good night's rest, even with the home Continuous Positive Airway Pressure machine designed to help her, and that she is exhausted pretty much all the time. She breaks down in tears in your office, telling you that she feels ashamed, frustrated, and hopeless about ever improving her situation, and she doesn't understand how she could have managed to raise three children, serve her community, and build a thriving business, and yet she can't manage to accomplish "this one thing"—that is, attaining and maintaining a comfortable weight. Your heart goes out to her, and—carrying an extra 20 pounds yourself after twenty-five years of practicing medicine—you understand her frustration. The ensuing conversation with Ms. Smith puts you ten minutes behind schedule, and your heart sinks with the expectation that the two of you are likely to have a similar discussion the next time she returns to your office.

In spite of their best intentions, after having the same conversations over and over for many years, some clinicians can't help but heave a mental sigh of frustration or feel a flicker of annoyance. We very much want to care and feel compassion for our patients struggling with eating and weight concerns, but after years of repeating our best advice without coming close to achieving the desired health outcomes we or they wish for, what we often feel is exasperation and despair, which cannot help but spill over into our treatment of the very patients who look to us for help and hope.

Unfortunately, these disheartening feelings, when combined with our rampant, undeniable cultural prejudice against fat and people who carry a great deal of it, may sometimes find expression in the form of weight bias and weight stigma (defined as making negative assumptions about health, motivation, or worthiness, solely or primarily based upon how much someone weighs). Sadly, the medical literature tells us that these prejudices are all too common among physicians, residents, medical students, and other health care providers,[1] and that this adversely impacts patient trust[2] and compliance and "can impair the quality of health care delivery."[3] Although we cannot make it disappear overnight, by acknowledging that we may, by virtue of living in this culture, harbor weight bias, we can bring it out of the shadows and into the light of day to be understood and eliminated. We can then discuss how it has come about and how it impacts the way we treat our patients, and also how it makes us feel about ourselves to experience cynicism and burnout when our goal is simply to help our patients optimize their health.

As health care providers, we are weary of proffering the same old eat-less-and-move-more advice that seems to go in one ear and out the other. We are tired of hearing how hard patients have "tried" to eat healthier or become more fit, and saddened that their meager progress may not mean much in their overall health picture, particularly if those small advances are not sustained over the long term, as is most often the case. More than anything, we frequently feel burdened with the magnitude of a job we never signed up for when we chose a career in the health professions: convincing patients to eat more nutritiously, become more active, and take better care of themselves on a consistent, sustained basis. Our patients are overwhelmed with this seemingly insurmountable task, and, frankly, so are we.

## WHAT EXACTLY ARE DOCTORS' CHIEF COMPLAINTS?

### Ineffective treatment recommendations, even for patients who are high functioning and generally successful

Doctors and health care providers often feel exasperated and ineffective, as many of their patients, despite being talented, educated, high-functioning, productive members of society, become heavier and sicker with each passing year. Some of our patients own and run enormously prosperous businesses, outearning us by leaps and bounds. Some have successfully overcome obstacles and adversity in their lives that seem to us to be much more challenging than losing and keeping off weight. "Why is this so difficult?" we ask ourselves and each other. We worry about our patients and think, "If you could just eat more healthfully, exercise, and lose and keep off 10, 20, or 50 pounds, your diabetes, hypertension, and hip problems might improve, and you would likely feel better, maybe even live longer. You have enormous talent, drive, resources, and intelligence. What can I do to convince you to take better care of yourself and motivate you to change your lifestyle for good?"

### Inadequate training and ineffective recommendations

Health care providers who care for patients with eating and weight concerns face myriad frustrations in trying to get and keep their patients healthy. Armed with inadequate training in nutrition,[4] we follow the guidelines of our esteemed medical societies in recording and reporting each patient's weight and BMI at each visit. For patients whose BMI falls above "acceptable" parameters, we are trained to prescribe calorie restriction and exercise and, in "extreme" cases, weight-loss drugs and surgery. Each year, despite their efforts, the majority of our patients on the high end of the weight spectrum, who wish to eat less or more healthfully, fail to achieve lasting success, leaving us more and more discouraged about our abilities to help them.

At the same time, our medical journals continuously remind us that we face a national and worldwide "obesity crisis," and that despite the time, energy, and resources that we dedicate to managing the conditions that we are told are caused by excess fat, our patients' weight struggles only intensify with each passing year. Many of our patients suffer a decreased quality of life, days missed from work due to conditions related to metabolic dysfunction, and hours and hours of productivity and satisfaction lost to food obsession, dieting, depression, and despair.

**Responsibility without control**

Although we make the argument later in this book that weight in itself is not the sole cause of all our higher-weight patients' health problems, there are certain medical circumstances in which patients with larger bodies and greater adiposity can face greater risks of a missed diagnosis, in the case of adipose tissue or body habitus compromising imaging quality,[5] or complications during and after anesthesia and surgery.[6] Metabolic derangements associated with obesity, poor nutrition, and chronic inflammation can compromise wound healing and recovery.[7] Undiagnosed obstructive sleep apnea often worsens with increasing BMI, and this can lead to dangerous desaturation before, during, and after surgery, particularly with narcotic use in untreated patients.[8] Higher-weight patients are at greater risk of blood clots and wound separation in general,[9, 10] and weight-loss surgery in particular entails unique risks in those who undergo this intervention.[11, 12]

**Maximally invasive, minimally effective options**

Speaking of surgery, over the past several decades, the medical establishment has concluded that if diet and exercise are not effective in achieving weight loss, then perhaps weight-loss medications and surgery will be. The side-effect profile and safety considerations of weight-loss medications have led to several being withdrawn from the market. The side effects and failure rate attendant to bariatric surgery serve as another source of frustration for surgeons and primary care physicians alike, as research indicates that 20–30 percent of postsurgical patients start to regain weight within two years, continuing to struggle with untreated emotional eating and body dissatisfaction.[13] We, as health care providers, know that we must be missing something important, when patients lose weight after bariatric surgery, then gain it back, despite their bodies having been *anatomically altered*. We cannot help concluding that there must be a better way to help these patients achieve lasting success.

### Pediatric Considerations: More responsibility without control

In pediatrics, doctors face even graver considerations. According to the Centers for Disease Control and Prevention, "Childhood obesity has more than doubled in children and quadrupled in adolescents in the past 30 years."[14] Our medical societies and peer-reviewed publications admonish us that if we do not take action, our children's generation may not outlive their parents, due to the adverse health consequences of obesity.[15] Obesity has been described as "an epidemic disease that threatens to inundate health care resources by increasing the incidence of diabetes, heart disease, hypertension, and cancer."[16] We are desperate to help our young patients, to put an end to this present and future misery, to prevent the impending health-related disaster that we are told is happening before our eyes and outside of our control.

And yet the options available to our pediatric patients, when calorie restriction and increased activity fail to deliver the sustainable weight optimization that we are told is required for health improvement, give us great pause. How can a child or adolescent truly consent to the available weight-loss medications whose side effects and long-term effects are still largely unknown? Is it appropriate to surgically alter the gastrointestinal tract of a youngster who will have to live with the consequences of that decision (including altered eating patterns for life) before he or she is even old enough to truly appreciate or evaluate the long-term repercussions of such a choice? Isn't it worth trying additional and more intense psychology-based measures prior to treating children who have high weights with invasive anatomical alteration, as though they were merely smaller versions of adults? Their brains, psyches, and bodies are not like those of their adult counterparts, and yet we in medicine are confronted with studies and guidelines from well-intentioned experts recommending bariatric surgery for our young patients.[17, 18]

Promoting weight-loss surgery and medications of questionable long-term efficacy and safety without investigating all available alternatives amounts, in our opinion, to metaphorically trying to push a boulder up a mountain with one or two fingers rather than using both hands. For some patients, surgical or pharmaceutical interventions may truly be their only hope to avoid metabolic disaster and certain death, despite the risks, and each individual must be treated by his or her personal physician on a case-by-case basis. For the vast majority of patients, however, such drastic (but too often minimally effective) corporeal interventions might well be avoided by focusing on building a psychological foundation for ending emotional and dysregulated eating. This means addressing the eating-related psycho-emotional issues and subconscious internal conflicts (often fueled by diet failures) that plague many of our patients with high weights and dysregulated eating patterns *before* taking more drastic measures.

Brain food for providers: What is your rate of success in helping your patients of size, who are dissatisfied with their weight, attain a healthy body and lifestyle that feels good to them? What other approaches, beyond calorie restriction and more exercise, have you recommended to them? Which approaches have been most and least successful? What strategies would you like to know more about that would help you further, given your time and practice constraints?

Despite the compelling medical explanations for why our patients (both young and old) might benefit from attaining and maintaining a "healthier weight," the calorie-restricted diet and exercise recommendations that we are trained to recommend ultimately fail to result in sustained weight loss for the vast majority of people. Studies show that, although most diets result in weight loss in the short term, the recidivism rate (or relapse and weight regain to even more than the pre-diet starting weight) is astoundingly high.[19] Furthermore, as we discuss in Chapter 3, a growing body of evidence indicates that deprivational dieting behaviors, particularly in childhood, may lead to bingeing, compulsive and/or disordered eating, and ultimately, weight gain—immediately, or even years later.[20, 21]

How frustrating that our best advice, the very recommendations that our medical societies and peer-reviewed publications promulgate, often results in abject failure, dangerous weight cycling, and despair in so many of our patients. How frustrating that we are doing the best we can and still failing dismally to help our patients succeed. Moreover, we, as health care providers, too often find ourselves in the same sinking boat as our patients: out of shape, sleep deprived, snacking non-nutritiously, stressed out, and foregoing exercise despite the fact that, more than anyone, we should know what is required to stay healthy and fit. Is it really fair to ask our patients to do what we haven't been able to achieve ourselves? There has to be a better way.

There is. Upon further reflection, many practitioners and researchers in the medical field have begun to wonder if there isn't a missing piece of the eating-weight puzzle. All of the daily small decisions that patients make about self-care, eating, and exercise take place *outside* of our offices and hospitals. Yet their frustrations and failures become ours when they return for appointments without having achieved the results that they, and we, desire for them. They believe that our advice is failing them and, thus, that *we* are failing them. And we might even subconsciously conclude that they are failing *us*. There's more than enough frustration and blame to go around.

### WHAT IS IT THAT WE'RE DOING WRONG?

We give our patients directives (sometimes even coupled with scare tactics, shaming, and threats), in order to motivate them, but we don't provide them with *effective* tools to sustain their motivation to eat better, exercise more, and care for themselves well and consistently. Their time with us is limited. Assuming they have the skills to eat well and take care of their bodies when they haven't been able to do so consistently in the past makes no sense. Without sufficient support, skills, and understanding of themselves, when destructive internal monologues, irrational impulses, and day-to-day stresses wear them down, the pressure of the ingrained habit to seek food for comfort or distrac-tion will nearly always win out. It is in these moments that our patients need our very best advice and our most effective tools to help them think, eat, and act in their own best interest. "Eat less, move more" just doesn't cut it.

### ALL TOO TRUE—BUT THEN, WHAT DOES CUT IT?

Until recently, effective strategies, as applied to eating, weight, and health struggles, have been largely missing from our medical training. Fortunately, the fields of psychology (particularly the psychologies of eating and of suc-cess) and motivational theory have produced exceptional tools that will enable our patients to understand why they don't take adequate care of themselves consistently, assume responsibility and accountability for their health, and feel empowered to think and behave in a way that promotes sustained well-ness. We maximize patients' chances of success when we help them learn and implement more empowering and effective psychological strategies, so that they can feed themselves well while maintaining internal motivation and a constructive mindset outside of our offices. Much less physically invasive, and without the side effects and morbidity of some of the behavioral, medical, and surgical alternatives just discussed, a psychology-based approach provides practitioners with useful tools and strategies that build patients' emotional intelligence, internal motivation, self-efficacy, and resilience, promoting the kind of consistent, sustainable behavior optimization that drives lasting wellness. These lessons, tools, approaches, methods, and strategies will hopefully reshape both clinicians' and patients' perspectives toward engaging in a more psychologically oriented, success-promoting approach to resolving eating, weight, and health concerns for good.

Consider this: What if our patients are not unaware, unmotivated, or lazy? What if they desperately wish to follow our advice but don't realize they're conflicted about implementing it and don't have the skills even if they were unilaterally gung ho? The truth is that many patients with eating and weight concerns are often reminding themselves of our recommendations for health improvement (and may be beating themselves up for their lack of consistent adherence) multiple times per day, living in an exhausting state of shame and anxiety over the present and future consequences of their "failure" to take better care of their health. The truth is that eating, food, and weight issues are incredibly complex, involving much more than the physiologic effects of a simple nutrition and exercise regimen for the body and far more than an earnest desire for wellness.

---

Brain food for providers: Was your medical training adequate preparation for you to work with patients who have overeating problems? If not, why not? What training would have better prepared you? What training or partnerships would help you be more successful now, given your time, clinical focus, and practice constraints?

---

## ARE YOU SAYING THAT PATIENTS' EATING AND WEIGHT CONCERNS ARE OUR FAULT?

No! As physicians (especially those over 30), most of us are poorly prepared to treat eating and weight concerns.[22] Rather than blame ourselves for our shortcomings in serving patients with weight struggles, we must understand that our training simply has not kept pace with new insights and research concerning motivation, eating, self-care, and weight.

Just as we have moved from viewing alcohol and drug addiction as moral issues to recognizing them as medical and biological ones, it's time to start thinking about eating problems not as moral failings or the result of a weak character but as biopsychosocial-emotional conditions that are multifaceted. Most of us received zero training in the psychology of eating, motivational theory, self-care skills, and personal development. Recent research suggests that these subjects are of critical importance in effectively treating patients with eating and weight concerns.

We maximize patients' chances of success when we help them learn and implement more empowering and effective psychological strategies, so that they can feed themselves well while maintaining internal motivation and a constructive mindset outside of our offices. Much less physically invasive, and without the side effects and morbidity of some of the behavioral, medical, and surgical alternatives just discussed, a psychology-based approach provides practitioners with useful tools and strategies that build patients' emotional intelligence and self-efficacy, promoting the kind of consistent and sustained behavior optimization that drives lasting wellness.

## ARE YOU SAYING THAT I NEED TO LEARN A WHOLE NEW SKILL SET IN ORDER TO HELP MY PATIENTS?

Right about now, we suspect that some of you might be thinking, "Don't I have enough to do without adding this time-consuming, touchy-feely, psychological mumbo-jumbo to the mix? How am I going to learn this psychology stuff well and fast enough to be of help to my patients with everything else I have to do?" Don't panic. We understand your trepidation and that you're already feeling overburdened and maxed out. With ever-increasing pressures for efficiency and speed in the practice of medicine (particularly in primary care, where patients typically present for "weight-loss" advice), physicians barely have time to adequately address medical conditions that may be immediately life threatening, much less explore the arguably less pressing, but no less essential, psychological underpinnings of eating and weight struggles.

Furthermore, the time spent by physicians in investigative or motivational interviewing and individualized emotional- and food-management counseling, which might get to the root of maladaptive eating and activity patterns, is often not remunerated. In the current climate of reduced reimbursements for medical care, it may seem overwhelming and unrealistic to dedicate precious time to implement a more cutting-edge, individualized, biopsychosocial treatment approach.

---

Brain food for providers: How are you feeling about learning new strategies from the fields of eating and success psychologies and motivational theory that will help your high-weight patients achieve their health goals?

---

The good news for doctors and health care providers is that the relevant material is relatively simple to learn and to implement once you understand why it is so important to the patient who struggles with overeating, regardless of his or her weight. Furthermore, more and better resources are emerging so that we as physicians do not need to have all of the answers for our patients in order for them (and us) to experience the success that has eluded them in the past. What providers *really* need to know (and what this book will teach you) is how to initiate productive, constructive discussions with patients on how they can implement strategies and practices that are successful for the long term. Our job is to collaborate with a motivated patient and, equally, to encourage a relatively unmotivated one.

Moreover, how clinicians *define the problem* for themselves and for their high-weight patients is critical to successful treatment. For some patients, weight struggles are genetically based and for others, they are simply the result of over-dieting for decades. However, in our experience, "weight" problems in many cases are actually rooted in what we call dysregulated eating and ineffective self-care, problems which must be resolved before patients can achieve consistency in the health-promoting behaviors that actually generate improved outcomes in physical and psychological health metrics.[23, 24] "Dysregulated eating" means eating when not hungry and not stopping eating when full or satisfied. Dysregulated eating involves lack of attunement or mis-attunement to appetite cues, misreading emotional discomfort as food craving, and inattentiveness to the act of eating which results in an inability to know when enough is enough. If health care providers are treating patients for "weight" problems, which are really dysregulated eating problems, how will our patients ever make progress?

We hope you're not thinking, "Eating disorders, what do I know about eating disorders? Isn't that the domain of psychotherapists and dieticians? Haven't I got enough on my plate as it is?" For the most part, when we speak of eating problems in this book, we're not referring to anorexia nervosa or bulimia nervosa. We're talking about eating mindlessly or emotionally due to stress, distress, avoidance, or boredom and not knowing when, or not being able, to stop eating or not start. Some dysregulated eaters might meet criteria for binge eating disorder, which will be discussed in more detail in later chapters. However, many of your patients who are living at a higher weight than they would prefer are simply overeaters, mindless eaters, emotional eaters, and compulsive eaters—in short, dysregulated eaters.

Engage in any of these behaviors often enough and, voilà, you have a "weight problem," a term, by the way, that does not accurately define what's going on with these patients, because, for many, the problem actually stems from one or more skill deficits in awareness, self-care, self-efficacy, and/or self-regulation that impede the consistent, sustained implementation of healthy lifestyle behaviors. Fail to address emotionally based eating and self-regulation problems as such, and you have a patient who appears to engage in "self-sabotage" and "lack of adherence" to the "treatment plan." Obviously, something is very wrong with this picture, and that wrongness is based in blaming the patient and defining the problem narrowly as one strictly of weight, when true health and wellness is about so much more.[25]

If you are ready to accept that most of your patients are desperate to attain a comfortable and healthy weight that reflects a balanced, healthy, self-directed life, but are continually undermining themselves due to subconscious internal conflicts and suboptimal life skills, read on to learn more about how patients really feel inside and outside of the doctor's office. If you do now or ever have struggled with your size or with eating dysregulation, and believe your struggles affect your ability to successfully treat patients with weight and eating concerns, our goal is to help and support you in your efforts for improved health. If you know that what you've been doing to help your patients attain and maintain healthy eating habits hasn't been working as well as you and they would like, and if you are ready for some simple psychological strategies to turn your work around, you've come to the right book.

Brain food for providers: Do you make assumptions about what type of person a patient is based upon his or her body habitus? How much of your frustration is based upon how ineffective your "diet and exercise" advice seems to have been in helping your patients maintain improved health in the long term? How much is due to your own feelings of failure and ineffectiveness in achieving success as defined by weight loss?

Providers, try . . .

1. Accepting that you are not a failure because your patients do not lose weight or keep it off after you have given them diet and exercise instructions, weight-loss medications, or they have had bariatric surgery.
2. Recognizing that the missing key to success with patients who overeat lies in the mind. We have been trained to recommend ineffective and incomplete strategies. If we can learn all that we did in our professional training, we can also incorporate approaches that harness the power of the mind-body connection and how it relates to food.
3. Telling yourself that you are perfectly competent to acquire new skill sets to help you and your patients succeed with resolving their eating and self-care problems.
4. Remembering that you are not responsible for implementing all of the elements of a successful eating or fitness approach for your patients.
5. Recognizing that nonjudgmental provider-patient collaboration is the most effective model for resolving eating and weight concerns and sustaining results.
6. Resisting the urge to be impatient with yourself for all you believe you need to know about the psychology of eating and reminding yourself that you will learn slowly like we all do, the way you did in medical, nursing, or other professional school.
7. Ignoring the urge to lecture patients about diet and exercise when you become frustrated that they're not changing quickly enough—or at all—and telling yourself that you are doing the best you can to help them and that they are doing the best they can to help themselves.
8. Learning how to ask questions that inspire awareness, introspection, compassion, understanding, and, ultimately, change. More on this skill set will be presented in future chapters.

# Why Patients with Eating and Weight Concerns Are Frustrated

## (Can't Doctors Trade in Their Stethoscopes for Magic Wands?)

- What it often feels like to live in a body on the higher end of the weight spectrum
- What makes higher-weight patients uncomfortable in medical settings
- How to stop the blame game between provider and patient
- What patients want out of their provider-patient relationship
- What providers and patients need to focus on to improve their relationship

If doctors are frustrated with failing to meet their goals of helping patients eat more healthfully and attain a comfortable weight, that frustration is nothing compared to that of their patients, many of whom have been on more diets than they can count. It's not as if people with high weights don't know that they're large. They have mirrors, buy clothes, listen to and read the news, and have families and friends who encourage them to be healthy and fit. Is there really anyone left in this country who doesn't recognize that thin is in and fat is out, and that this narrow (pun intended) standard isn't going to change any time soon?

In the next chapter, you'll learn why the well-intentioned efforts of doctors, health care providers, and patients alike haven't resulted in permanent weight loss, enhanced self-efficacy, or increased body acceptance for the majority of our patients. For now, we ask that you put stock in either your own experience with dieting and weight regain or what you've observed about others—patients included—circling through this revolving door.

For now, our goal is to help you understand what concerns patients bring to each medical visit aside from a desire to leave the office feeling better than they did when they came in. Those of you who never have considered what visiting the doctor may be like for higher-weight patients might be very surprised to learn what's going on inside their minds. If you're a doctor or health professional, you've probably been focused, quite naturally, on what's going on with your patient's body, and less so on their hearts and minds. Moreover, you might find surprising all the things we'll describe about what and how these patients feel as they enter, sit in, and leave your office.

Not to worry. After all, you may not have thought much about this subject before. Commendably, you want to learn, which is why you picked up this book.

Brain food for providers: What judgments about higher-weight patients are crowding out your curiosity to learn more about them? What judgments about yourself are barriers to being curious about your own reactions? Gently remind yourself to stay curious and let go of judgments about yourself or your patients. Be compassionate with your own imperfections, and you'll have an easier time being compassionate with those of your patients.

## HOW DO PEOPLE WHO HAVE HIGH WEIGHTS AND EATING PROBLEMS FEEL?

Readers who struggle with eating and weight concerns will no doubt recognize our description of feelings you've experienced with your doctor or health practitioner. You may have had experiences strikingly similar to the ones we describe, finally feel validated by our words, grow angry or sad, or sink into despair that the doctor-patient relationship will never change when it comes to eating or weight concerns.

You may be shocked at the intensity of your rage, which has built up over the decades and has had no place to go. Maybe you tried to tell your doctor how you felt, but he or she didn't have time to listen or didn't try to understand. Maybe you stopped going to certain health practitioners who were highly skilled because you left your appointments feeling miserable about yourself or were scared that if you stayed for one more minute, you would bite their heads off and say something which would bias them even more strongly against you. Or perhaps you're ashamed that you never stood up for yourself and now feel riddled with anger or regret.

Patients and providers, we urge you not to judge your feelings. Simply observe that these are your emotions for now and that they are neither wrong nor right, but true expressions from the heart. Patients, pay special attention to your desire to blame yourself for "being fat" and feeling "difficult to treat," for thinking of yourself as a failure, and for feeling more compassion for your poor doctor who has to treat "over-sized" you than you do for yourself. Understand that viewing yourself negatively due to your size or weight is an assumption that keeps you feeling down on yourself. With self-compassion, patience, and practice, you will learn to view yourself in a more positive, accepting light and, from that place, your chances of successfully reaching your eating goals will improve markedly.

---

Brain food for patients: What are you feeling right now? What judgments are crowding out your curiosity to learn more? Gently remind yourself to stay curious and let go of judgments about yourself or your providers. Find the place in your heart that has compassion for yourself no matter what your size, weight, or eating problems are.

---

## SO, WHOSE FAULT IS THE "OBESITY CRISIS," THE DOCTOR'S OR THE PATIENT'S?

Let's stop the blame game right here. Patients have been doing their best and so have doctors! We know this may be a mind-blowing statement, but it's based on one of the basic tenets of psychology which goes like this: We're all doing the best we can all the time *and* sometimes our best at that moment isn't good enough.

Both parts of this axiom are true. We *are* doing our best at all times *and*, sadly, often our best just doesn't cut it. This may be a difficult concept to wrap your mind around. Psychotherapists spend a good deal of time explaining this principle to clients, followed by lengthy and intense debates about its validity. Eventually, clients do come around to this way of viewing humanity.

Understanding this concept is crucial because it generates compassion and validation, acceptance, and humility. When you accept that people (including yourself) are doing the best they can do all the time, due to previous experiences and current internal resources, it moves you to acknowledge their (and your) humanity. It validates that sometimes our best is woefully inadequate precisely because we are imperfect human beings. The point is that holding these two thoughts gives you permission to fail, yet also says that you can strive to do better, which, for doctor and patient alike, is what this book is all about. There is hope and powerful potential in the decision not to give up, no matter how challenging a task appears.

Now, let's move on to the focus of this chapter: why patients are so frustrated with the doctor-patient relationship as it relates to dealing with their eating and weight concerns. Here's what we've learned and want to share with you from the patient perspective.

### In general, heavy patients are uncomfortable stepping on the medical office scale and, therefore, dislike and wish to avoid this ritual

We all know that hopping on the scale at the doctor's office is de rigueur. Believe it or not, many patients start thinking about this anxiety-producing aspect of the appointment weeks or days before an office visit. They dread standing on the scale because they either know what they weigh and are miserable about it or don't wish to know because it will make them miserable due to what their doctor will have to say about it.

To them, a scale is not a neutral mechanical object. It's a *shame machine*. As it's busy doing its calibrating, it might as well be announcing, "You are a big, fat person and bad for it," or "Have you no shame weighing what you do?" While the nurse records a number—137, 201, 314—the patient is experiencing herself as bad, defective, and a huge disappointment. Because of their internalized shame, critical self-talk, and societal stigma, it can feel awful for some patients to confront what they weigh. There is powerful, emotional work that patients can do to improve their self-talk, including not judging themselves harshly when they step on the scale[1] but, in the interim, making that most-feared number public knowledge is like shouting out their deepest, darkest secret disgrace to the world. It is a recipe for despair that can actually derail patients' ongoing efforts at wellness for days, weeks, months, or even years.

Some brave patients may request not to be weighed and see where that gets them. Other patients may tell the nurse that they do not wish to know what they weigh and turn around so that they're not facing the numbers on the scale but away from them. However, even making these requests draws attention to their large size when, at the point of being weighed, all they want to be is invisible. The whole business is embarrassing and feels stigmatizing enough to keep patients away from entering a doctor's office and receiving much-needed medical attention. According one study, "A total of 19% of participants reported they would avoid future medical appointments and 21% would seek a new doctor if they felt stigmatized about their weight from their doctor."[2] This is a frightening truth: some patients may not come to appointments if you insist on weighing them.

**Patients are fed up with deprivation and denying themselves the pleasure of foods that are considered "too high-calorie" and "too high-fat" for them to eat**

Whether life has been one long diet or they've jumped on and fallen off the diet bandwagon dozens of times, it is not easy for people to watch others eat yummy foods knowing they're *verboten* to them. Or, more accurately, to know that the price they'll pay for a few, fleeting moments of mouth-watering ecstasy will be far steeper than it is for the majority of folks. Generally, "normal" eaters say yes and no to food more or less in balance. They can eat a little bit of high-calorie or high-fat food and stop before they go overboard. People with eating problems (which usually morph into weight dissatisfaction) are different.

For whichever combination of biological, environmental, and psychological reasons, they are unable to say yes and no to food in balance. Maybe it's due to all-or-nothing thinking (to be discussed later in this book), so that they're either off "forbidden" foods or eating nothing but them. Maybe it's because they're genetically programmed to have a high-weight set point—that is, our (more or less) biologically determined weight. Or maybe it's sheer habit from food being their only comfort in childhood. Or possibly it's because they stopped listening to their own feelings and appetite signals decades ago when a parent or doctor put them on a diet and, over time, with repeated dieting, they lost the ability to sense hunger or satiation. Or they were taught to believe that their worth was measured by their success in attending to the needs and concerns of others at home, in school, at work, and in relationships, and therefore disconnected from their own desires, both physically and emotionally, and turned to food for solace and reward.

Whatever the reasons, it's time to stop making a moral issue of it by insisting that patients lack self-discipline and self-control. This premise is false and you will learn more about why later in this book. The truth of the matter is that it's painful and frustrating for patients to walk around feeling as if they'll be forever on the outside looking in, their noses pressed up against the glass watching other people eat what they believe they must deprive themselves of. They end up feeling like they're damned if they do eat something they crave and equally damned if they don't. Sometimes saying no just gets too hard and feels too unfair and so they throw in the towel and say, "The hell with it," and then seek solace by eating whatever they want, forgetting about good intentions as well as bad consequences.[3] Honestly, when that kind of tension builds up and they lack the self-awareness and skills to intervene, the inevitable response is that they end up lost in the all-too-short-lived pleasurable gastronomic moment.

**Patients bring to every doctor's visit their deeply felt helplessness, hopelessness, self-contempt, and despair about their body size**

In most cases, these patients are not actually helpless. There is usually (but not always) something, even one small thing, that they can do to take care of themselves better to become healthier. But, sometimes not. Sometimes all they can do—what they've been struggling to do for decades—is to avoid gaining any more weight than they already have. The truth is that they often are not totally helpless, but relentlessly feel as if they are. Anyone and everyone can tell them not to feel that way, but they needn't bother. We all feel what we feel—until we learn to feel another way.

Telling patients that they shouldn't feel helpless because rationally they're not is a waste of your time and energy. They feel powerless, not necessarily about the present and losing weight, but about keeping it off so they won't be back in a doctor's office having this same conversation a year or two from now. Trust us, they remember every diet they ever began, their high energy and bright hopes, the power they invested in the conviction that this time would be different, the initial outpouring of support from family, friends, and coworkers, and the dreams of a slimmer future and what that would mean for them.

And they remember, even more clearly, how nothing worked, or at least not for the long term. All their diet failures, whether long ago or recent, are etched in their memories and take up a wide swath of mental real estate. They loom far larger than happy memories of success, love, achievement, and other pleasures. Take note: These deeply felt, perceived failures are often the defining feature of these patients' lives and the basis of their identity: I am doomed to be fat no matter what I do. I Am A Fat Failure. Forever.

You may wonder why we include both the terms "helplessness" and "despair" in describing how these patients feel. Think of it this way: Despair is helplessness on steroids. It is believing not only that you cannot do anything about your situation right now but also that you *never* will be able to. Despair is giving up the dream or the fight, surrendering to any future possibility of weight loss because you're never going down that road again. Despair is giving up trying because you believe you cannot bear another weight loss and regain, that you'd rather be fat and stay fat than taste thinness and have it stolen from you by the greedy gods of appetite.

---

Brain food for patients: Which of the above-mentioned problems have you experienced in a doctor's office? Which has been most difficult for you? Say aloud or jot down what you would like your doctors to know about what you've experienced and how you felt.

---

**Patients often have lost and regained hundreds of pounds**

Most of them know they can lose weight, or, at least, they know they *used* to be able to do so. They've done it, more than once, sometimes two or three or eight times. Do the rest of us have any idea of the discipline that is required to lose 100 or maybe 200 pounds by dieting? That's like trimming off half of yourself in the most excruciating fashion, day by day, meal by meal, mouthful by mouthful. So many people complain about being unable to lose those "darned last 10 pounds," while many patients have lost ten or twenty times that much and sometimes have kept it off for months or years. If anyone is an expert on weight loss, it's the person who's gone down three or five sizes more than once. How many of us can imagine the deprivation and determination that took?

While others—doctors, family, friends, coworkers—look at them and think, "Why can't they lose weight?" people who are currently deemed fat but who've lost large amounts of weight are wondering, "Why can't I keep weight off? Why do I always gain it back? What is *wrong* with me?" This is a different experience than most of us will ever have: to succeed and fail, then succeed and fail again. The problem isn't weight loss, but rather weight regain. Many in the medical establishment are looking at these patients as folks who've done nothing, while they're looking at themselves as folks who've done everything they were supposed to do and still failed. And how do you think that makes them feel?

Many of these "yo-yo dieters" also know that each time they've gone through the ordeal, the gradient has become steeper. The same push to shed mega pounds leads to less reward each time, and often, sadly, more effort does not reap commensurate success. Rather than previous dieting making it easier to give a repeat performance, it actually makes the process harder.

Ironically, "yo-yo dieters" see themselves as compliant patients: They've done exactly what doctors have asked—dieted and dieted and dieted again—and they still can't make the number on the scale go down or stay down. Paradoxically, doctors often view them as noncompliant because they haven't kept weight off. These opposing views get in the way of having productive conversations about what can be done. And, truly, if the only answer to weight loss is dieting and patients have done this ad nauseam, then they and their doctors are at an impasse, unless they're going to consider weight-loss drugs or surgery.

**Patients are tired of hearing and believing that if they wish to be fit, they will have to suffer and punish their bodies, because, in this culture, "fit" means "thin"**

Don't get us started on programs like *The Biggest Loser* and *Extreme Weight Loss*. These programs are nothing like reality—at least none we've experienced. How many of us would embark on an endeavor that we know will be long on pain and short on pleasure? Okay, other than suffering through the sleep deprivation endured in medical school and residency. It's not that patients don't want to be fit. They do, sometimes more than anything else in the world. But, let's face it, it's harder to move a large object than a small or medium-size one. It's often difficult for many patients to walk, never mind jog. We're not making excuses for them. It *does* take more effort. And they worry about what to wear to the gym, especially to the kinds of clubs where hard-bodied folks are decked out in fashion-statement workout wear. They worry excessively about what people will think of them, that they'll look silly, that others will view their efforts as too little too late, that they will be laughed at and pointed at (because it's happened before), and that it will take so long to get fit that they'll be old or dead before they succeed.

### Even if they're eating better and exercising, if their weight doesn't drop, patients of high weight feel like failures

Because this culture is so fat phobic and weight obsessed, if these patients do manage to eat more healthfully, consume smaller portions, and reduce mindless or emotional eating on a consistent basis and don't lose weight, or lose it quickly, they still feel like failures. If they're fortunate, their lab numbers improve and they cling to that small blessing to prove that, in fact, they *are* doing what they were told to do and desperately want to do: take better care of themselves. If their lab numbers don't budge *and* their weight remains the same, even if they are on the right track and engaging in healthy lifestyle behaviors, who will cheer them on?

Basically, they feel like huge disappointments if they're not getting healthier quickly or quickly enough. It's not like our culture encourages slow and gradual change. No, we're all about to do it now, do it right, and get it done. More is better than less (except in the fat body department) and faster trumps slower. Where do we ever hear the message that slow is better than not at all? Whoever champions the gradual, yet enduring, solution?

Mostly, people feel like failures because they are frustrated when they are eating healthfully and exercising and still can't shed much weight. They also feel like failures because most are unremittingly hard on themselves. (You will learn more about this personality trait in Chapter 4.) Even when others, doctors included, praise their small achievements, they often see *only* what they didn't do and have yet to do, not what they've already achieved. And, they can be very convincing about their failures unless the people around them adamantly refuse to allow them to see themselves as walking disasters and, instead, zealously point out their everyday successes, however minor.

---

Brain food for providers: When you look at your heavy patients and hear their weight-loss and regain histories, do you see someone who's tried or someone who's failed? Do you feel pressure to help them change quickly or can you champion the most minimal improvements in behavior?

**Most high-weight patients are aware that their bodies may not fit the current cultural ideal and feel demeaned, shamed, and infantilized when doctors tell them that they need to lose weight**

Patients get rightfully annoyed when they're told that their BMI or weight is too high as if they had no idea this was so, as if they mistakenly thought they were Ken or Barbie, as if this were some sort of breaking news bulletin. They have mirrors and buy clothes and are perfectly capable of comparing their bodies to other people's bodies (which they are usually obsessed with doing, much to their chagrin, unless they've given up completely due to despair and depression). If anything at the doctor's office will enrage them, it's being told in whatever way—sternly or kindly, patiently or impatiently, with concern or aloofness—that they are "overweight" and need to lower the number on the scale.

Upon hearing doctors tell them that they're "overweight," or have gained weight recently, what many really want to say (and rarely, if ever, are bold enough to do so) is "Really? No kidding? Gee, I had no idea. I'm shocked, but so glad you mentioned it." Why don't they share these thoughts? Well, because most of them would rather put on 20 more pounds than offend a doctor whom they often see as an authority figure, whom they want to like them and care about them, and whom they need desperately when they have medical problems. So, when they're told they're overweight, they nod and smile and make it seem like doctor and patient are on the same page. Nothing could be further from the truth.

Imagine these perspectives: Either patients have totally given up on the idea of losing weight because they have come to believe from experience that nothing will work for them or they tell themselves that they are so fat that it would take them several lifetimes to slim down. Alternatively, they may have spent the time since their last doctor visit eating more moderately and healthfully and haven't seen the number on the scale budge. Whatever the case, hearing that they're "overweight" will almost always compound their frustration and make a bad situation a great deal worse. At best they will feel enormous shame—and at worst they'll feel enormous shame.

**Patients with eating and weight concerns, like everyone else in the world, hate to be lectured**

No one likes to be lectured. On one level, especially if they genuinely like their physician, most patients recognize that their doctor means well. Really they do. Therefore, they will most likely sit meekly through the lecture that the doctor is none too happy to be giving in the first place. So, here you have a doctor who feels helpless but duty bound to give the Lose Weight Or Else 101 (or 202 or 303) lecture to an audience of one who feels more ashamed and disempowered with every word that's uttered. Or, alternately, an audience of one who tunes out the blah-blah-blah completely because he or she has heard it a gazillion times before, so often that he or she can almost repeat it verbatim.

When patients are lectured by even the most well-meaning doctors, they only *feel* smaller. It doesn't actually help them *get* smaller.

### Knowing their doctors are unhappy with them, patients fear upsetting them more by asking questions

These patients may already feel unlikable, or maybe even unlovable, because of their large size. So very many of them were teased and bullied in childhood or adolescence for their girth. They are often desperate to be liked and highly sensitized to even the tiniest whiff of disapproval. They are so sensitive that they experience a kind of paralysis when they are lectured about their weight so that they just sit there and tune it out or wish they could disappear on the spot. Afraid they might antagonize the doctor further (beyond what they fear their largeness already has done to cause disfavor), they clam up and forget or ignore the questions they came in to ask.

Not asking these important questions does two things. First, it increases their sense of helplessness, powerlessness, and the power differential between doctor and patient. Second, it leaves patients at a disadvantage because they forgo finding out information that is crucial to taking good care of their health. Such lack of information may lead them to not doing what is necessary to manage their health problems and to putting themselves at further disadvantage at their next visit, a vicious cycle if ever there was one.

### Patients become upset when doctors say or imply that every ailment they have is due to their poor eating habits, lack of fitness, or weight

No other complaint by these patients about doctors (except perhaps mandatory weigh-ins) is as anger producing as being told (or having it intimated by their providers) that every physical problem they experience is due to their weight. Perhaps not all, but many patients understand that weight puts stress on their hearts and joints, may make surgery more difficult, and may put them at risk for certain serious diseases. But they also know that their thin and average-weight friends visit doctors with symptoms similar to theirs and that many physical ailments have little or nothing to do with weight.

Between the two of us, we know thin, average-weight, and heavy people who have spinal stenosis, knee and back problems, sleep apnea, acid reflux, high cholesterol, hypertension, cancer, and a plethora of other physical conditions. The fact is that sometimes a cigar really is just a cigar. This doesn't mean that a high weight might not aggravate some conditions, such as arthritis/degenerative joint disease, obstructive sleep apnea, high blood lipid levels, and inflammatory illnesses, but it doesn't necessarily cause the problem and losing weight won't necessarily eliminate it, even if we assume it might help. Patients want to know and trust that whatever physical ailments they bring to their doctors' office will be viewed from a neutral, nonweight-biased perspective and taken seriously.

On a related matter, patients become frustrated when they make an appointment to talk about, say, a sore throat or a pain in their groin, and the discussion ends up being about their unhealthy diet and lack of exercise. If doctors overfocus on patients' weights, they're going to be less effective in treating the range of conditions we all have. And their patients may trust them less and avoid making appointments until they are in dire need of medical attention. These patients want to know that they will be looked at as patients first and fat second (or maybe third or fourth), not the other way around.

Brain food for patients: What do your doctors do that makes you feel demeaned or shamed? What do they do that makes you feel they are in your corner? How do you usually handle upsetting interactions in a medical office? How will you take charge at your next appointment and ask the questions you want about any of the medical problems you have?

**Some patients fervently wish their doctors could fix their eating problems and are frustrated and angry when they can't**

Though some people insist they don't find doctors helpful, most of us are enormously grateful for the medical skill and knowledge that keeps us healthy. We know we are! Rightly or wrongly, we expect doctors to make us feel better, heal our physical problems, and ease our suffering. This is in part due to our views of their expertise and authority (e.g., valuing their education, training, and experience) and also due to the way some doctors present themselves as omnipotent.

We are not here to debate how we got to this point in the history of medicine. We're trying to explain the mixed feelings that patients with eating and weight concerns may have about how doctors interact with them. These patients may not even be in touch with their conflicting feelings. After all, physicians are amazing healers for so many conditions and diseases. Most of us leave a doctor's office with the appropriate diagnosis, prescription, set of exercises, or the right protocol to follow to feel better. We recognize that we are so dependent on doctors to keep us disease free and healthy that we sometimes forget that they are not magicians (even when they act as if they are), but mere mortals.

When it comes to lifestyle changes, doctors can do little more than make recommendations, but patients sometimes demand more: bariatric surgery, the "right" weight-loss diet, the newest drug or supplement that advertisers swear will take away their appetite and slim them down. Because physicians can actually cure and heal so much of what ails us, it can be enormously frustrating for these patients that their major concern above all else—their eating or weight—cannot actually be fixed by their physician because the small, daily, incremental decisions and choices that determine lasting success or failure happen outside the clinician's office. And because the underpinnings of their "weight" problems actually may be based on their genetics or their difficulties managing the *rest* of their lives and their conscious and unconscious beliefs about food, eating, and many other things.

**Patients who have eating and weight concerns are insulted when their doctors lack compassion for them and, in fact, may be judging them for their high weight**

These patients are often very, very, very, very sensitive to judgments about their size. They sometimes see slights where none exist, take things personally which aren't meant that way, and think that other people are as down on them as they are down on themselves because of their weight. The truth is that sometimes they're right and sometimes they're wrong. Studies show that many doctors, reflecting the society we live in and the perceived realities of the enhanced risks that excess fat creates for patient care, do hold a bias against large-size patients.[4, 5] Their prejudice may slip out via their words and tone when they don't even realize it.

However, doctors also may be perceived as judgmental when they don't mean to be. It can be very difficult for heavy people to discern when they're being viewed pejoratively, because they're so super-sensitive on the subject and because they have often been judged harshly and cruelly in the past. They are used to being shamed, stigmatized, harassed, bullied, teased, criticized, and demeaned. Society does it all the time implicitly and explicitly.

There's no question about it. Folks make a fat-phobic remark, but, when called on it, insist they were just joking around. Moreover, people who have high weights are ridiculed on TV and in the movies, as if they had no feelings at all! Weight is truly the last bastion for prejudice. It is the job of all of us—fat, thin, and average weight—to be part of the solution to this injustice.

Rightly or wrongly, people look to their doctors not only due to their intelligence and skill but also for compassion. Most of us assume that physicians chose their calling to help people and, therefore, we expect them to be compassionate. The fact is, some doctors with terrible interpersonal skills are brilliant diagnosticians and others are only fair to midland practitioners with the most caring bedside manners. Most people can shrug off the former, but doing so is often very difficult for patients who so desperately want acceptance at their large size, to not feel judged, and to believe that doctors are in their corner.

### Patients may get confused about the difference between being cared for and being controlled, which leaves them frustrated with what they want from their doctors

An internal conflict that is not well understood outside of psychological circles is the issue of care versus control. This means that we are often confused about whether someone is caring for us or trying to control us. This common psychological quandary is hardly limited to patients or folks with eating or weight concerns. But, the fact is, for this population, it can be extra difficult to discern what a doctor's motivation is: Is he or she telling patients to do something eating- or weight-related due to genuinely caring about them or is the doc trying to control their behavior to feel less helpless and more successful? How can patients tell the difference? And what can they do if doctors don't seem to really care, but just want them to do what they advise because it's expedient and they have no other constructive approaches to offer?

This care-versus-control conflict comes up frequently with people who weren't cared for well in childhood. Starting back then, parents and teachers told all of us what to do, insisting that we comply with their advice or demands because they cared about us—and because it was good for us. Well, sometimes they did care and sometimes they didn't—and maybe it was good for us and maybe it wasn't. What if they regularly wanted us to do things because it made their life easier or made them feel better? What if their directives really were more about their needs (the unhealthy parent-centered household) than about ours (the healthy child-centered household)?

So, when patients who encountered rigidly controlling and demanding parents, teachers, coaches, or other authority figures are told to do something about their weight, even by a caring physician—even by a caring anyone—they may perceive that this individual is trying to control them. This happens more than you would think and is part of transference, a generally unconscious process by which, in adult life, we ascribe to others the personality traits of our parents or other significant people in our early lives. Some patients are so wary and resentful of being controlled, especially about their weight and particularly if they've had eating problems or were made to diet in childhood, that they think all authority figures (and even nonauthority ones) are trying to control them even when this is not the case. The slightest hint of pressure to do this or not do that may cause an automatic fight or flight response when they feel they're being manipulated. This psychological dynamic crops up often during interactions with authority figures, not just doctors, and can totally derail the doctor-patient relationship unless it is well understood, addressed, and resolved.

A doctor might really worry about a patient's poor eating habits, but express his or her feelings in such a cold or authoritarian manner that the patient feels not cared about but controlled. Doctors must be highly attuned to their tone of voice and choice of words in order to sound as far from controlling as they possibly can. Additionally, it's vital that patients reflect on whether they often feel controlled when people express caring and the desire to help them. These patients would benefit greatly from acknowledging if they have issues about being controlled and then working to resolve them, especially in the doctor's office. They need to recognize that not everyone in authority is out to manipulate and dominate them and that their physicians may genuinely care about what is in their patients' best interest.

**Patients of higher weight are often uncomfortable when asked to disrobe and required to wear a medical dressing gown**

One additional reason for discomfort is that patients may be wildly uncomfortable when health care practitioners request that they undress for examinations. Most patients with high weights are terribly ashamed of their bodies and many don't ever look in the mirror because they can't bear what they see. So, imagine what it's like to have a virtual stranger, whom they expect will be judging them harshly for their size and shape, see them up close and extremely personal. Moreover, imagine what it's like to put on a dressing gown that you fear will be or actually is way too small for you. Truth be told, there are patients who avoid going to the doctor simply because they must undress to be examined.

---

Brain food for patients and providers: What mixed messages do you get or give in the doctor-patient relationship? How can providers best express caring? How can patients share concerns when they feel controlled or don't feel cared about?

---

After reading these first two chapters, doctors, health care providers, and patients will hopefully have a greater understanding of the barriers that have prevented them from communicating effectively about health and enjoying a collaborative, productive relationship.

If you are a person on the higher end of the weight spectrum, we hope you now feel understood regarding what it has been like for you to make medical visits—and maybe even why you chose to stop going to them. If you are a doctor or other type of health care provider, we hope you now have an insider's view of what it is like to receive medical care in a large body.

Are we saying that every heavy person in this society has experienced everything we've written in this chapter? Of course not. But, the truth is that there is a wide gulf that has continued to widen between patient and medical provider as our culture has become more fat phobic and weight obsessed. Our intent is for providers to start looking at their higher-weight patients in a more respectful and compassionate manner and work with them more constructively and compassionately so that both patient and provider can achieve success.

Providers, try . . .

1. Phrasing your wish or expectation as a request such as, "How would you feel about . . . ?"
2. Explaining—briefly, rather than lecturing. The first time we say something, we're giving new information. After that, it's called nagging.
3. Training your staff to ask patients how they feel about getting weighed and disrobing and respect their wishes whenever medically appropriate or feasible.
4. Reducing pressure on yourself to "fix" your patients, even if the pressure is coming from them.
5. Paying attention to how you feel about patients who have eating and weight concerns and seek to feel compassion for them.
6. Noticing patient's body language which may mean they're anticipating a lecture, are uncomfortable with what you're saying, or wish to speak.
7. Validating patients' smallest efforts in a positive direction—what they're doing well—and avoiding mention of what they're doing wrong or have yet to do.
8. Putting yourself in patients' shoes and consider what it's like—without judgment!—to be a person who is large in this culture. Be humbled! And empathize, empathize, empathize.

Patients, try . . .

1. Relaxation exercises (deep breathing works wonders) before going to doctors' appointments that you anticipate might be stressful.
2. Watching out for conflicting feelings about doctors—wanting them to fix you, but knowing you must fix yourself; wanting to do what they say, but hating being told what to do.
3. Making a list of your questions before your appointment and giving a copy to the doctor at the start of the visit.
4. Telling providers if you're sensitive about your weight, especially about disrobing or being weighed, and speaking up if you feel he or she is shaming or putting you down.
5. Describing to providers in writing your entire dieting and weight-loss history, all your successes and failures, especially what works for you and what doesn't.

6. Sharing your hopelessness over your eating or weight concerns and requesting referrals to registered dieticians, Intuitive Eating counselors, fitness trainers, wellness coaches, and psychotherapists who are appropriately trained and specialize in eating problems.
7. Viewing the provider-patient relationship as a collaboration, with them doing their part and you doing yours.

# 3

# How Diets Kill Motivation and Make People Fatter

## *(Who Knew?)*

- What a typical weight-loss diet consists of
- The science behind why weight-loss diets fail for the long term
- How diets promote weight gain
- The reasons people hate dieting
- How to recognize the dysregulated eater and why dysregulated eating often underlies overeating and weight struggles

Let's be clear: When we talk about dieting, we're talking about intentionally restricting calories, food types, or quantities for the sole purpose of shrinking our bodies. We're not speaking of diets prescribed for food allergies or intolerances, or those which are necessary for specific medical conditions such as kidney or liver disease or endocrine considerations. In the medical field, we have been taught (and reminded countless times) that putting patients on a calorie-restricted diet is the best initial strategy to promote weight loss—provided, of course, that patients stick to the diet. The truth is that both our professional experience and current research on weight loss tell us that, for most patients, *calorie-restriction dieting does not lead to permanent weight loss*, nor does focusing on weight or BMI as an outcome result in improved physical or psychological health.

In fact, as we will discuss in this chapter, quite the opposite is true: Dieting is actually a proven risk factor for weight gain, weight regain, disordered eating, and, ultimately, weight cycling,[1, 2] which contributes to the chronic diseases that weight loss is purported to prevent![3, 4] A substantial amount of recent evidence demonstrates that becoming healthier and preventing disease may be less about weight loss and more about lifestyle and self-care strategies than we have been led to believe.[5] In this chapter, we'll review the many reasons that the "diet for weight loss" strategy, which we as clinicians have been trained to believe in and promote, may be not only ineffective but, worse, downright counterproductive,[6, 7] particularly if dietary composition is not optimized. These reasons relate to the metabolic, biochemical, psychological, and behavioral consequences of calorie restriction, which (lest we forget) the body perceives as a form of starvation.

The authors both have been on diets galore and had friends and patients who've embarked on them, and if you'd asked us or them about the desired result of those endeavors, our collective answer would be: to lose weight, of course. The problem is that the goal is far more appealing than the process endured to reach it. It's a good deal easier to cozy up to the idea of dieting than to actually stick to one for any length of time. Here's the definition of the verb *to diet*: "Restrict oneself to small amounts or special kinds of food in order to lose weight."[8] Seriously, how alluring do "small amounts" and "special kinds of food" sound—*for the rest of your life*? Depressing, that's how. If weight-loss diets worked permanently, well, okay, we might try to put up with feeling deprived and denied pleasure. But if they're going to make us miserable *and* fatter, really, what's the point?

In her book, *End Emotional Eating*, Jennifer Taitz, Psy.D., reminds us, "If you define yourself by your weight, you may restrict your food, and restricting food often leads to overeating."[9] To help you understand what food restriction really does to us, let's look more closely at the current medical recommendations and the latest research when it comes to dieting for weight loss.

## WHAT IS THE MEDICAL ESTABLISHMENT'S CURRENT RX FOR HIGH-WEIGHT PATIENTS?

According to the 2013 AHA/ACC/TOS Guideline for the Management of Overweight and Obesity in Adults, calorie-restricted diets and increased exercise are the recommended initial interventions of choice for patients who are found to be "overweight" or "obese."[10] Regarding calorie-restricted diets, the guidelines state:

> Prescribe a diet to achieve reduced calorie intake for obese or overweight individuals who would benefit from weight loss, as part of a comprehensive lifestyle intervention. Any one of the following methods can be used to reduce food and calorie intake: a. Prescribe 1,200–1,500 kcal/d for women and 1,500–1,800 kcal/d for men (kilocalorie levels are usually adjusted for the individual's body weight); b. Prescribe a 500-kcal/d or 750-kcal/d energy deficit; or c. Prescribe one of the evidence-based diets that restricts certain food types (such as high-carbohydrate foods, low-fiber foods, or high-fat foods) in order to create an energy deficit by reduced food intake.[11]

This advice from the medical establishment is not new. Calorie restriction for weight management has been recommended for decades. Scores of diets are promoted each year with the common theme being that if you follow the diet and restrict your food intake, you will lose weight.

Yet, despite millions of attempts to implement these guidelines by countless well-intentioned providers and patients, as individuals and as a society, we have failed to lose weight or, more discouragingly, have failed to lose weight without then gaining it back—and then some. In fact, according to Linda Bacon's book, *Health at Every Size: The Surprising Truth about Your Weight*, "extensive evidence documents that attempts at dieting typically result in weight cycling, not maintained weight loss. Weight fluctuation is strongly associated with increased risk for diabetes, hypertension, and cardiovascular disease, independent of body weight."[12] Here's the typical pattern: Deciding that they need to lose weight for medical or other reasons, patients start a restrictive diet in which they eat markedly less or eat "more nutritiously" for a certain amount of time. Initially they feel elated, virtuous, righteous, and strong—until they start to feel cranky, tired, resentful, and deprived. If they fail to shed pounds on one diet, or if they lose weight in the short term but it creeps back on, they become frustrated, blame themselves for being failures, and seek another diet or recommit to the one they were on.

Providers blame patients for being lazy, noncompliant, or lacking willpower (a form of weight stigma), and the diet industry makes out like bandits, reaping billions from "repeat customers," who fervently hope that the answer to their weight-related woes lies in the next fad diet or nutritional guideline. Sounds addictive, doesn't it? According to data by Marketdata Enterprises, a market research firm that specializes in tracking niche industries, Americans spend upward of $60 billion annually to try to lose pounds, on everything from paying for gym memberships and joining weight-loss programs to drinking diet soda.[13] The US diet industry spends $59 billion per year to hook and rehook us on their plans and programs.[14] However, an analysis of twenty-five weight-loss studies found that dieting was actually a consistent predictor of weight *gain*.[15] And rather than improving motivation and health-related behaviors, internalized weight stigma and body shame have been shown to be associated with a reduced health and well-being.[16]

When patients and their health care providers give up on the "diet and exercise" recommendations as "ineffective" or "unrealistic," the pharmaceutical and medical device industries are waiting in the wings to profit from our habitual reliance on medications and surgery to "cure" what we cannot seem to fix without them. These interventions are not without side effects and risks of morbidity and mortality.[17] Not only that, but, like diets, pills and surgery also fail to address critical, underlying biological, behavioral, and psychological factors that drive dieters to overeat in the first place. As one of Karen's patients said post–bariatric surgery, "My stomach may have shrunk, but it can still fit a Snickers bar into it."

## WHAT'S WRONG WITH DIETING?

Since the 1980s, and likely long before, experts have suspected that restrictive dieting not only fails to result in lasting weight loss but actually leads to weight gain over the long term. In her groundbreaking book, *Secrets from the Eating Lab*, Tracy Mann, Ph.D., University of Minnesota professor, research scientist, and expert in the psychology of eating, diet, and self-control, opens Chapter 1 with a simple pronouncement: "Diets don't work." Mann goes on to describe in vivid detail the evidence that calorie restriction does not result in lasting weight loss for most people. Among other research, she cites a two-decade-old 1991 study that states, when it comes to the long-term results of dieting behaviors, "it is only the rate of weight regain, not the fact of weight regain that appears open to debate."[18]

In 2007, Mann and her colleagues at UCLA published a study titled *Medicare's Search for Effective Obesity Treatments: Diets Are Not the Answer.*

They reviewed all of the available randomized controlled studies that followed dieters for at least two years after the diet began and found "little support" to recommend dieting for sustainable long-term weight loss. "From one third to two thirds of participants in diets will weigh more four to five years after the diet ends than they did before the diet began."[19] The authors go on to explain that this less-than-optimal result is likely a low estimate, because these studies are often biased (by virtue of being weight-loss industry supported), terminated too early to see the full extent of weight regain, confounded by a high dropout rate among those who fail to lose weight or fail to keep it off, and are subject to other flaws like allowing participants to self-report their weight by phone or e-mail.[20] The conclusion that Mann and her colleagues arrived at may surprise you. "It appears that dieters who manage to sustain a weight loss are the rare exception, rather than the rule. Dieters who gain back more weight than they lost may very well be the norm, rather than an unlucky minority. . . . The benefits of dieting are simply too small and the potential harms of dieting are too large for it to be recommended as a safe and effective treatment for obesity."[21]

---

Brain food for providers: What has been your personal experience with diets—yours, family members', friends', colleagues' success? What has been your professional experience? Have you assumed that people fail diets or that diets fail people?

---

### WHY DON'T DIETS WORK LONG TERM?

Researchers have known and health care providers have suspected for decades that restrictive dieting does not result in either sustained weight loss or sustained improvements in physical or mental health for the majority of people. There are several proposed reasons for this. First, experts estimate that our genes control approximately 70 percent of how much we weigh, what's called our set point range.[22] Second, restrictive dieting is perceived by the body as a form of starvation, and within it multiple collaborative and redundant mechanisms have evolved to prevent weight loss and favor weight regain, in order for the human species to protect the genetically and biologically determined set point and survive in the face of famine or food scarcity.[23]

When calories are restricted and weight is lost, appetite and food cravings escalate, increased levels of ghrelin, GIP, and pancreatic polypeptide promote feelings of hunger, and decreases in levels of leptin, insulin, peptide YY, amylin, and cholecystokinin blunt fullness signals.[24, 25] At the same time, metabolism slows to conserve energy. Third, as fat is lost, so is lean muscle tissue. Levels of fat storage enzymes increase, and it becomes more and more difficult to sustain weight loss even with fewer calories, both because the body becomes more efficient at storing calories and because energy levels decrease.[26]

Even worse, with the loss in lean muscle mass as a result of calorie restriction, when weight is regained (as, studies show, it inevitably is), body composition changes, resulting in a greater percentage of body fat compared to the percentage prior to starting the diet, a concept known as "fat overshooting."[27] This is the body's way of saying, "Hey, I get it. I'd better prepare in case there's no food around for a while." This relative loss of fat-free mass, or lean muscle mass, further contributes to a more sluggish metabolism and a reduced need for calories to maintain the same weight as before the diet.[28]

Scientists believe that the physiologic basis for weight regain after dieting is mediated in part by hypothalamic control over appetite and energy expenditure (as a response to hormonal signals from adipose tissue, the GI tract, and other peripheral sites), and in part by physiologic changes (including those in regulation of appetite, substrate metabolism, and energy expenditure)[29] that encourage weight regain and interfere with maintenance of hard-won weight loss.[30] Also known as yo-yo dieting, weight cycling is the natural result of many dieters' attempts to lose weight through restrictive eating practices, and it may be far more dangerous than previously thought. Far from being an indicator of a failure of a dieter's willpower, weight cycling actually represents the body's natural biologic and psychological compensatory mechanisms that seek to keep it alive during periods of starvation.

It is now scientifically accepted that this all-too-common weight fluctuation places the chronic dieter at risk for diabetes, hypertension, and cardiovascular disease, *independent of body weight*.[31] And lest you think that only people of high weight are at risk, a recent study by Dulloo et al. demonstrates that the risk extends to *persons of normal weight* who engage in dieting and weight-cycling behaviors, a trend that is on the rise as the cultural ideal of thinness clashes with our admittedly obesity-promoting environment.[32] What has become clear in recent years is that dieting most often leads to weight regain, with many dieters regaining more weight than they lost and damaging their bodies and self-efficacy in the process.[33]

According to Linda Bacon, Ph.D., who is an expert in psychology, eating disorders, exercise science, and metabolism, the author of *Health at Every Size: The Surprising Truth about Your Weight*, and the creator of the Health at Every Size program that has been demonstrated in NIH-supported research to help people improve their health without dieting or focusing on weight loss, "Not one study has ever shown that diets produce long-term weight loss for any but a tiny number of dieters."[34] Moreover, Bacon points out that dieting has been shown to interfere with the body's innate weight regulation system, through biological, psychological, and behavioral mechanisms.[35]

So, not only do diets fail to result in permanent weight loss and result in weight gain over time, but "extensive evidence" cited by Bacon also demonstrates that restrictive dieting practices "typically result in weight cycling, not maintained weight loss." Bacon corroborates Dulloo et al.'s findings that it is actually this weight fluctuation itself that is "strongly associated with increased risk for diabetes, hypertension, and cardiovascular diseases, independent of body weight."[36]

It is important to note, however, that weight loss (or prevention of further weight gain) achieved through healthy lifestyle habits and consistent exercise is a different story. According to research cited by Bacon, "active people are much healthier than sedentary ones, regardless of weight. Exercise can cure, prevent, or minimize most of the major chronic diseases and disturbances, including diabetes, insulin resistance, hypertension, high cholesterol levels, cancer, digestive disorders, circulatory disorders, etc."[37] The importance of regular physical activity to overall health is one of the foundational principles of Lifestyle Medicine, and a Lifestyle Medicine–based approach, with a focus on wellness, rather than weight, *per se*, can be transformative for patients who struggle with dysregulated eating behaviors. We will discuss this approach in detail in Chapters 7 and 8.

We understand that hearing the facts about diets' failures may be a bitter pill to swallow. If you remain unconvinced about the drawbacks of prescribing calorie-restricted diets for patients of high weight, consider this advice from a prominent registered dietitian and eating disorders expert. According to Evelyn Tribole, M.S., R.D., "Dieting increases your chances of gaining even more weight in the future, not to mention increase your risk of eating disorders, and body dissatisfaction."[38] Tribole and coauthor Elyse Resch, M.S., R.D., F.A.D.A., C.E.D.R.D., write extensively about the association between dieting and weight gain, as well as the dangers of dieting to overall health, in their 1995 landmark book, *Intuitive Eating*. It is now in its third edition, and recent research continues to support their admonitions that (calorie-restricted) dieting is not the answer to overweight, even combined with exercise.[39, 40]

As health care providers, we are confronted with evidence from respected experts, numerous research studies, and our own clinical (and often personal) experience that for the vast majority of people, dieting for long-term, sustained weight loss is ineffective. And we are beginning to realize that chronic dieting may actually contribute to the diseases (type 2 diabetes, hypertension, heart disease) that it is supposed to prevent, by promoting "weight cycling"[41] or repeated weight loss and regain. And yet, for a number of obvious and not so obvious reasons, we, as health care providers, are still instructed to recommend dieting, along with exercise, as the primary tool for weight loss in patients with "elevated" BMIs or high weights. This lack of attention to the biochemical, psychological, and metabolic consequences of restrictive dieting for susceptible individuals can be a recipe for rampant frustration, as we know from our clinical experience.

Perhaps this is due to our not believing that we have an effective alternative to offer our higher-weight patients, and that not encouraging food restriction will result in their eating without restraint and gaining even more weight. Perhaps it is because we know that even if dieting did work, most of our patients would fail to implement these behaviors consistently over long periods of time. Restricting food and calories by trying to exert self-discipline and willpower over the biological imperative to eat is fighting a battle just waiting to be lost. Patients despair, and so do we. We watch our patients, friends, and family members (and maybe ourselves) fail at dieting, succeed temporarily, but then regain the weight, or seem to not pay attention to what they are eating, and we are riddled with frustration and feelings of futility. Unfortunately, many of us then conclude that our patients must be unmotivated because they do not persist with engaging in the behaviors that we recommend.

In addition to the metabolic and hormonal considerations outlined above, there is, however, another important cause for the long-term failure of diets: the psychological reasons that diets fail. These psychological considerations may well hold the key to helping troubled eaters permanently mend their relationship with food, regulate their eating, and improve other wellness-related behaviors. We will revisit this topic in Chapter 5, but for now, we present you with the psychological reasons that diets fail, which those of you who have struggled with food and the scale know all too well.

## WHAT ARE THE PSYCHOLOGICAL AND BEHAVIORAL CONTRIBUTORS TO DIETING FAILURES?

Often overlooked by the medical establishment, but equally important as the physiologic changes induced by calorie restriction, are the very real psychological considerations that derail weight loss when a person is dieting. Dieters feel deprived and often become apathetic, depressed, and obsessed with food. Dieting causes stress,[42] which increases circulating cortisol and predisposes the dieter to inflammation, vascular damage, hypertension, insulin resistance, and the accumulation of abdominal (visceral) fat.[43] Stress also negatively impacts sleep, which, as any medical resident will tell you, often results in increased food intake to compensate: traditionally in the form of tater tots deep fried in the hospital cafeteria fryer, consumed in the dark to stay awake during morning radiology rounds. But we digress . . .

After they get over the initial heady surge of excitement about the idea of losing weight, the three major reactions that most chronic dieters have to restricting food by type or quantity are overfocusing on what they can and can't eat, feeling deprived, and experiencing cravings that lead to obsessions about food that border on stalking. Note that it's the idea of losing weight that patients love, not the actual process of doing it. That's like wanting to be a home-run hitter while dreading batting practice, or dreaming of winning the Nobel Prize in physics without learning about quantum theory. It's hard enough to reach reasonable goals when we love what we're doing and practice our hearts out. It simply is out of the question when you don't really want to do the things you must do to reach your goal.

### Overfocusing on food in the quest for weight loss

Even as we are dieting, we desperately wish to take the focus off what goes into our mouths. At the same time that we want to eat fewer calories or grams of sugar, we also want food to mean less to us, to move off center stage in our lives. But, inevitably, dieting puts it smack dab right in the spotlight. Funny how our minds work: When we tell ourselves not to think about food, it's just about *all* we can think of. Psychology tells us that by directing ourselves *not* to do something, rather than forget about it, we are more likely to keep thinking about the thing we're not supposed to do. Try a quick, simple experiment to prove this theory: Keep telling yourself not to touch your hand to your face, and what do you end up thinking about? Touching your face, of course.

Note that there's a world of difference between a hyperfocus on food and what's called mindfulness, which involves putting all your attention on appetite cues when your body says it's hungry and savoring the experience during the entire eating process. When we hyperfocus, forbidden food and the satisfaction that we believe it will provide become something divine, and we long for it like a lost lover to whom we've given magical powers. When we hyperfocus on eating healthfully, we erroneously think, "Eating this will make me thinner." When cravings overpower us and we don't care that what we're eating may harm us, we think, "Eating this will make me happy."

Both of these cognitions miss the point of eating: the food in front of us. Longing for the future goal, be it thinness or happiness, rather than being present to the moment, we are anything but mindful about what we're eating. Mindfulness means thinking about nothing but the texture, smell, and taste of food while we're ingesting it, with no thought to what we ate yesterday or might eat tomorrow, or how any of our food intake is going to affect our weight. Mindfulness means thinking about how what we're eating feels in our bodies as we eat it. When we remove our attention from the present moment and the food that we are eating in it, we are likely to end up eating more because we are not present to the experience of pleasure, fullness, or satiation. Instead, we are focused on the goal (weight loss or happiness), and miss out on paying attention to appetite cues which will likely help us reach it. Ironically, we have the process exactly backward.

### Deprivation

Most people who restrict their eating to lose weight gradually experience an intense feeling of physical and emotional deprivation. Suddenly, life seems tremendously unfair and maybe even despairingly empty: we're on the outside looking in. Sometimes we fail to notice anyone who is also restricting his or her food intake and only take note of folks getting seconds at the salad bar, ordering scrumptious desserts (not stewed fruit, mind you), or eating our favorite dishes, which we fear will never again pass through our lips. We envy them and covet what they're eating, think they're lucky, or that life is unfair because we believe they can eat whatever they want and we can't. Irrational thinking, perhaps, but that's how the human brain works. Alternately, we may notice other dieters, those poor, unfortunate, sad souls who are also condemned to the Dieting Ring of Hell, the one that Dante failed to mention in *The Inferno*.

How sadly ironic that deprivation makes food restriction and denial feel almost noble. Like the men in Ancel Keys's famous starvation studies during World War II, we boost our spirits by sharing recipes, food fantasies, diet tips, pitfalls, successes, and downfalls, all the while trying to keep feelings of deprivation at bay by telling ourselves and each other that we're going to be successes because our culture reveres what we're doing.[44] We are so proud of the pain of self-denial. Sometimes this enables us to ignore the gnawing in our bellies and the light-headedness that makes us woozy, and other times we want to weep from how badly we want to eat "real" food or simply more of the foods we love. We may alternate among feeling hopeful, irritated, hopeless, superior, or sorry for ourselves. How we feel depends as much on what we didn't eat (that candy bar) as what we did eat (our third salad of the day), and the more diets we undertake, the more the deprivation grows. Our despair accumulates and eventually drives us to think and behave irrationally when it comes to taking care of our health.

### Food cravings and obsessions

When we deprive ourselves of foods we enjoy, in quantities that satisfy us (in other words, when we diet for weight loss), food is on our minds 24/7 and we spend much of our time absorbed in thinking about what we crave. Instead of filling out our income tax forms that are due next week, we're fixated on that key lime pie we baked for the grandkids who are coming over for lunch tomorrow. The funny thing is that we never really liked key lime pie and can't recall the last time we ate it—a year, maybe several years ago. But now we can almost taste the tartness, almost feel the lightness of the meringue dissipating on our tongues—and can think of nothing else.

Studies tell us that when we deprive ourselves of nourishment and calories, we cannot help but put them front and center in our minds. In the aforementioned classic study by Ancel Keys, a professor in the School of Public Health at the University of Minnesota, "thirty-six men volunteered to be starved for six months as a humanitarian act so that researchers could test the best ways to help starving people throughout the world." Eating researcher, Traci Mann, Ph.D., who cites this study in *Secrets from the Eating Lab*, says of it, "Although this study is always referred to as a starvation or semi-starvation study, I think of it as a diet study, because the men were allowed nearly 1,600 calories per day."[45]

Mann goes on to describe the study's results. "All sorts of things happened to the men during the study . . . but the most common *psychological* response was an obsession with food. Before the study started, the men had many interests. . . . But when the men were starving, the only thing they wanted to think about, or could think about, was food."[46] The obvious evolutionary reason that when we're deprived of calories, we obsess about food, is to keep us alive. Put in this context, our cravings and food obsession make perfect sense, but theoretical understanding does little to help us when biological imperative takes over and we want what we want when we want it. This obsession with food and eating, as Mann points out, "steals valuable attention from other activities, and the more preoccupying food thoughts dieters have, the more difficulty they experience thinking about other things and handling other cognitive tasks, [such as those related to memory and problem-solving]."[47] Thus, sadly, the life of the chronic dieter slowly shrinks as he or she becomes more focused on food, eating, body dissatisfaction, and the quest for weight loss, at the expense of living a full and balanced life.

Brain food for patients: What has been your dieting experience—positive or negative? Do you still diet and hope this time you'll be able to keep off the weight or have you given up on dieting? How do you feel about your doctor prescribing a diet for you?

## ARE THERE OTHER REASONS FOR ENCOURAGING PATIENTS TO AVOID DIETING?

Considering the biological imperative to eat in order to live, arbitrarily advising clients to cut down on food (even for constructive reasons), especially to eliminate specific food groups, and causing them to feel deprived and food obsessed doesn't make sense or mesh with reality. Moreover, deprivation and preoccupation with eating are only a couple of the troublesome reactions that dieters have when they restrict calories and give up foods they love. Does this mean that there's no alternative to dieting and that we're recommending that patients continue to eat as non-nutritiously, excessively, and mindlessly as they have been? Absolutely not. We're simply trying to provide a clear and comprehensive picture (should you be one of the handful of people in this country who have never dieted or who actually enjoy a lifetime of food deprivation) of what you—and your patients—are up against.

Beyond food deprivation and food obsession, dieting causes people to do three things: disconnect from natural, innate appetite signals; become disempowered, criticize themselves relentlessly, and feel like failures when they don't lose weight or as much as they'd like to lose; and engage in rebound eating and stop taking effective care of themselves all around.

### Disconnection from appetite

Dieting for a long period of time (long enough for significant weight loss to happen) cannot help but promote an almost total disconnection from appetite, the mechanism humans use to determine when, what, and how much to eat. Surely we as health care professionals don't want our patients to learn to override their appetite signals? Do we? We would posit that our common goal is to help clients reconnect to and recalibrate their ability to sense authentic hunger, recognize food cravings, savor true pleasure from food, and stop eating when they're full (a.k.a. having eaten a sufficient quantity of food so that eating more would cause physical discomfort) or satisfied (a.k.a. having reached a peak of pleasure, rendering eating beyond this point as less pleasurable).

Patients cannot and will not be able to achieve this "attunement" (as Tribole and Resch describe it in *Intuitive Eating*) through dieting, when every program or plan drags them further and further away from their natural appetite cues. Do you really want to teach your patients to give up the internal locus of control they were born with and, instead, substitute an external source (in this case, a restricted-calorie diet plan), which robotically and arbitrarily tells them when or what or how much to eat? When people are tuned into and use their own, natural, innate sense of how to respond appropriately to body cues, we call them "normal" eaters. The word "normal" is in quotes because each "normal" eater is unique. Some eat according to hunger and cravings by enjoying three hearty meals a day with no snacking. Others prefer consuming small amounts of food every few hours. There are among "normal" eaters, breakfast lovers and breakfast haters, people who snack before bedtime and those who eat nothing beyond the dinner hour, those whose hunger response, through repetition, has become regulated by the clock, and those who "skip" set mealtimes to eat only when hunger pangs prompt them.

What all these eaters have in common is that they're guided by appetite and by the four rules of "normal" eating: (1) eat when you're hungry, (2) choose foods you believe will satisfy you, (3) eat with appetite awareness and an eye toward pleasure, and (4) stop eating when you're full or satisfied.[48] Obviously this innate attunement teams up with good judgment, food availability, and other factors that lead us to eat or not eat. If we're planning to attend an early buffet dinner, we may consciously choose to have a light lunch. If we expect to be in a setting in which we might get hungry and food won't be readily available, we'll likely wish to bulk up beforehand to compensate. "Normal" eating doesn't mean simply relying on appetite and chucking our reasoning skills out the window. It means being aware of appetite at all times, relying on it most of the time, and self-regulating our behavior by making conscious (rather than mindless), deliberate, ongoing choices around food that reflect our commitment to eating in our best interests.

### Generation of self-criticism, disempowerment, and despair

Brainwashed as they are to believe that they have no self-control or self-discipline or are too uncaring about themselves to stick to a diet, when they fall off the wagon or don't lose weight (or sufficient amounts of it), dieters begin to feel deep disappointment in and criticize themselves. They look around and see friends and family (and celebrities) in different stages of dieting, most of whom are excited when they begin a new program or plan or ecstatic because they've lost a few pounds. TV programs are in the business of showing us, not the failures, but the successes. Commercial weight-loss programs are not required to share outcome data in their advertising, and the medical studies that promote calorie restriction for weight loss often do not follow dieters long enough to demonstrate the dismal truth about how few people sustain more than a two-pound weight loss or about the very real weight regain that does not seem to level off over time.[49] Given this lack of accurate, unbiased information about the inefficacy of dieting for weight loss, it is no surprise that most dieters wonder what's wrong with them or what they did wrong.

Mistakenly, they blame themselves for failing, rather than recognizing that the game was rigged from the start—that diets have failed them because such is the nature of chronic food restriction when up against a biological imperative. It's no good telling them that they should try harder or try again or that they didn't fail because they tried. They mistakenly believe that the number on the scale is all that matters: that people who lose weight are the success stories and people who don't can't help but feel like perpetual losers.

No matter how beautiful or handsome, wealthy or accomplished, adored or admired they are, many people who can't stick with or lose sufficient weight on a diet feel like failures. Moreover, it's difficult for them to compartmentalize their disappointment and distress, and acknowledge that the rest of life is good or even a great deal better than good. It's not fair—and they know this, which makes the sting of defeat so much harder to bear—but, for many, this failure at weight loss cancels out their successes at everything else. In this way, dieting undermines both patients' self-efficacy and self-trust in their ability to know what they need and take care of their bodies.

Disenchanted, demoralized, and despairing of ever having a positive relationship with food or their bodies, they too often retreat into comfort eating and gain back the pounds they've shed, and then some. It will be a while before they take any interest in the dieting process, and sometimes they give up completely. Let's be clear: this doesn't mean they don't want to be healthier. On the contrary, their failure or string of diet failures will continue to haunt them because they want to feel comfortable in their bodies so badly they can almost taste it. Only now, they're convinced that the comfortable body they want will always be beyond reach. Add to this the fat shaming and weight stigmatization that are so prevalent in our culture, along with the judgmentalism of the medical establishment that remains, sadly, less the exception than the rule, and it's no wonder that patients despair of ever succeeding in reaching their goals.

### Rebound eating and poor self-care

When people diet, initially they're on top of the world in spite of their self-denial with food. Suddenly they like themselves more and treat themselves as if they deserve health and happiness. They plan, shop for, and prepare nutritious foods, go for medical checkups, get to the gym as they've promised themselves (and you) they would, and generally take better care of themselves than when they were eating more mindlessly and less nutritiously. This happens because losing weight (or even the promise of losing it) gives them value in their own eyes (defining value in this way, is, of course, a huge part of the problem). They feel in control of their lives, powerful, positive, and forward looking.

But, when dieting doesn't pan out, all that feel-good self-care often comes to an abrupt halt. They may "forget" to plan ahead for meals and snacks, not bother keeping routine medical or dental appointments, stop exercising, and basically write off their health. One by one they give up their self-care behaviors. Disempowered and depressed, their self-worth plummets. What kind of person, they ask themselves over and over, can't stay on a diet and lose weight when the experts insist that it is the best course of action and when everyone else seems to be doing a fine job of it?

When they feel badly enough, to comfort themselves and give themselves solace, they eat, a concept referred to by Tribole and Resch as "food rebellion."[50] Or they eat because they're enraged—with everyone who told them they could get a handle on food and with themselves, because they can't do this one thing, which means more than virtually everything else to them. They eat to satisfy the cravings they have ignored so many times, to soothe their psyches after telling themselves (misguidedly) that they're pathetic incompetents at weight loss, and to punish themselves for their perceived failure. The word itself is like a giant billboard in their minds: You, Denise or Frank, you, you are a FAILURE!

We hope that the foregoing helps you understand and appreciate that restrictive dieting is not an effective or empowering treatment for people with high weights, or even for those of normal weight who wish to minimize their risk of weight gain. You might as well go ahead and advise them to diet—if you want them to gain weight and struggle with eating problems for the rest of their lives. The fact is that you haven't meant to do harm, but that's exactly what calorie-restrictive diets and a narrow focus on weight loss in the name of health promotion have been doing to your patients. Considerable evidence cited by Tracy Tylka, Ph.D., and colleagues demonstrates that this type of "weight-normative" approach leads to weight cycling, which is directly linked to diminished health, higher mortality, an increased risk of eating disorders, and internalized weight stigma, all of which can adversely affect sustained self-care behaviors and well-being.[51]

## WHAT EXACTLY IS DYSREGULATED EATING?

The unacknowledged truth that medical clinicians and even patients are often unaware of is that most eating problems are not attributable to laziness or to a lack of motivation and willpower. Dieting behaviors ultimately fail to lead to lasting weight loss because they do not address the underlying reason for food (ab)use and weight gain in the first place—that many people with "weight problems" use food to cope, avoid feelings, distract or self-soothe, and compensate for critical self-talk and disempowering beliefs, rather than for reasons of hunger, satiety, and pleasure, a concept known as "dysregulated eating." Dieting exacerbates this pattern, by the way, and we'll explain how. Although it is common to hear emotional or overeating labeled as disordered, we prefer the word dysregulated because we want people to eat "normally," in a regulated way.

Dysregulated eaters, who likely make up the lion's share of chronic dieters, use food for many purposes other than to satisfy hunger or cravings, and because of this, they fail to stop eating when they are physically satisfied. This is true whether they are dieting or not. They will overeat French fries when they are not on a diet and bean sprouts when they are. From hot fudge sundaes to roasted bell peppers, they overeat because they are using food to address, suppress, cope with, or avoid issues unrelated to physical nourishment. Dysregulated eaters will follow the diet you prescribe to the letter, restricting their intake and eating "virtuously" for days, weeks, or months, because they truly want to be healthy. But then one day a seemingly unrelated disappointment or challenge, or perhaps a small slip, such as eating an extra piece of low-fat cake, will launch them into a full-blown binge that leads them to eat to compensate for both the shame of the binge and the pain of past deprivation. This reactive overeating can last for days, weeks, or months on end, and results in tremendous shame, due to the dieter's internalization of cultural messages about overeating as an indication of laziness, sloth, lack of motivation, and character weakness. What might surprise you is that what looks like self-sabotage to both patient and provider may actually be a misguided attempt at self-care, and we will visit this concept in future chapters.

Given this reactive, unpredictable, and inconsistent eating behavior, it is not surprising that the dysregulated eater is often living above his or her body's preferred set point, or natural weight. Contrary to their own conclusions and to those of their health care providers, people who suffer from dysregulated eating are not unmotivated. *Far from it!* Many dysregulated eaters are highly successful and accomplished in virtually every other area of their lives. They are also not lazy. For some, much of their time may be spent actively attending to admirable health-promoting behaviors, such as shopping for fresh, local produce, preparing balanced, nutrient-dense meals for their families, and even exercising religiously.

What undermines dysregulated eaters is that, as Tribole and Resch point out in *Intuitive Eating*, when their lives become unbalanced, often even before they realize that anything is amiss, they turn to food to cope.[52] They restrict food, they binge on food, they celebrate with food, they obsess about weight, they repair despair with food. They reward themselves with food and they punish themselves with food. Food is their go-to source of comfort, consolation, relaxation, enjoyment, excitement, escape, and indulgence. They are like artists who paint with one color only, musicians who can play only one note. Their sole mode of expression is food. Unfortunately, it is also the source of their greatest frustration, sorrow, and pain. Food and eating occupy a central place in their lives and they regard it (often unconsciously) as far more than a necessary source of physical sustenance.

Imagine how such persons might fare when they dutifully act on your well-intentioned recommendation that they restrict their eating for the sake of their health. As much as they might desire to lose fat from their bodies and become healthier, they are psychologically in no position to sustain restrained eating when the inevitable obstacles inherent in being alive arise. There is not enough willpower in the universe to compensate for inadequate self-care strategies and ineffective life skills, including the ability to self-regulate emotions. Dietary restriction actually exacerbates the vulnerabilities common among people who use food for purposes such as self-medicating feelings, alleviating boredom, avoiding dreaded tasks, or celebrating life's events with an easy, inexpensive source of sweetness and temporary satisfaction.

Why would anyone use food in such a misguided way, you may wonder. The answer is that many dysregulated eaters lack effective self-care strategies and life skills that would prevent them from relying on food for a disproportionate share of their daily pleasure and comfort quotient. This attempt to use food to self-regulate may be their very best coping strategy. Food is cheap, plentiful, legal, and often tasty. Unlike overuse of drugs, alcohol, or other ways that people have been known to self-medicate, overeating to manage the vagaries of daily life does not have immediate negative consequences for others or for society at large. Using food inappropriately will not result in a citation for drunk driving and won't land you in court or in jail. Misuse of food is, on the whole, a pretty understandable coping mechanism.

But using food inappropriately or indiscriminately does have consequences, of course, including a higher weight than one might prefer and a gradual erosion of self-efficacy and self-trust. Regularly using food for reasons other than physical hunger can actually prevent dysregulated eaters from acknowledging and identifying their emotions and developing and practicing the skills to manage them. When we consider the psychological vulnerabilities of the dysregulated eater in the broader context outlined above, our well-intentioned advice to our patients to engage in calorie-restricted dieting "as a lifestyle change" now appears to be a truly counterproductive tool in the fight against unwanted fat.

Does it surprise you to learn that your patients might just be using a cheap, legal, tasty, comforting substance to self-medicate unmet emotional needs or compensate for inadequate life skills? Until those needs are acknowledged and self-care strategies and life skills learned to meet them in sustainable, health-promoting ways, all of the education on ways to restrict calories, burn calories, substitute "healthier" foods, and find alternate sources of entertainment are doomed to failure. This simple fact may be the least studied and least addressed, but possibly most important consideration that undermines success for our patients in normalizing their eating. For a detailed explanation of dysregulated eating and the self-regulation deficits and internal conflicts that underlie these patterns, we refer you to Karen's book, *Starting Monday: Seven Keys to a Permanent, Positive Relationship with Food.*[53]

Lest you think that "dysregulated eating" is only a problem for people with psychological dysfunction, you should know that many psychologically "healthy" people, and particularly many high achievers, eat in the absence of hunger as a strategy to meet a variety of (sometimes unconscious or unacknowledged) needs. People use food to get through their day, bridge the afternoon slump, cope with stress, put off unwanted tasks, comfort a bruised ego following an argument or a perceived slight, exert control over or take a break from a seemingly or suddenly unmanageable life, relax, or soothe the sense of overwhelm when everything in their day feels like work. The (often unacknowledged) unmet needs that food may be used to try to satisfy include the need for rest, a break (also known as work-life balance), self-care, self-esteem, self-regulation, nurturing, confidence, meaning, a higher purpose, intellectual stimulation, reciprocal relationships, fun, pleasure, passion, body acceptance, and even excitement.

In light of all of the needs that people use food to try to satisfy, it is not surprising that so many highly successful, educated, and motivated people (including many physicians and health care providers) struggle with eating and weight concerns. Within this context, it might be easier to understand that weight struggles do not indicate a lack of motivation or willpower for the vast majority of people. Rather, battling with the scale more often than not indicates a lack of effective self-care strategies and skills for regulating feelings, thoughts, and behaviors and turning reactions into responses. Restricting calories or food intake without attunement to appetite or emotional or physical needs is an ineffective method for achieving either a comfortable weight or improved health and well-being for the long term. Ongoing attunement and self-regulation are essential if the dysregulated eater is to achieve and maintain a comfortable relationship with food.

## HOW DO I KNOW IF MY PATIENT IS A DYSREGULATED EATER?

If your patient is living above his or her natural weight and frustrated about it, struggling with weight cycling, or is at a normal or even low weight, but constantly dieting, you may be treating a dysregulated eater. Of course, sometimes "normal" eaters have high-weight set points and you will want to be careful not to confuse high weight with necessarily having dysregulated eating or body dissatisfaction. Additionally, dysregulated eaters are often perfectionistic high achievers, who maintain lofty standards for themselves. They judge and criticize themselves harshly for any perceived shortcoming, and often engage in categorical or "all-or-nothing" thinking. They sometimes tend to be rule followers, which may explain why they abuse food, rather than more illicit substances. Alternately, they may hate rules and yo-yo from low to high weight because they are only willing to follow food guidelines for so long.

These well-intentioned patients are not trying to make themselves fat or sick, nor are they out to frustrate you, their dedicated health care provider. Rather, they are choosing the best way they have found (so far) to deal with not only their life circumstances, but also their feelings and thoughts about them, which, by the way, are often unconscious, and dysregulated eating helps keep them that way. We'll learn more about the personality traits of the dysregulated eater in Chapter 4, but, for now, it's sufficient to understand that these patients are doing the best they can, and our society's judgmental attitude and admonitions to simply "eat less and move more" only add fuel to the fire of their entrenched shame, frustration, and despair.

Now that you know more about how diets fail patients, both psychologically and physically, are you ready to give up prescribing them for patients with eating and weight concerns, in favor of more beneficial and less harmful strategies to promote health? We hope so. In future chapters, we'll present alternative tools and methods for addressing these concerns in a more effective, empowering way that can help patient and professional alike feel—and be—more successful.

---

Brain food for providers: How often when treating patients with high weights have you thought about diets promoting deprivation and food obsession? Have you viewed reasons given by patients for not wanting to diet or failure to adhere to diets as excuses or do you recognize the validity of their perspective? Do you feel frustrated and wish you had better advice for them?

---

Brain food for patients: How has feeling deprived around food as well as food obsessed affected your ability or willingness to diet again? What would you like physicians and health care providers to know about the food and diet experiences you've had and how they affect your eating today?

---

Providers, try . . .

1. Taking a diet history of your patients—asking about the number and types of past dieting experiences they've had, along with questions related to their body image—and really listening to what they have to say.
2. Reading between the lines about what patients say about dieting and what you sense they actually feel about—that is, that they like the idea of dieting but not the day-to-day process of engaging in it.

3. Asking patients to tell you about the times they've comfortably eaten according to appetite—what we call following the rules of "normal" eating regarding hunger, cravings, eating with awareness, and stopping when full or satisfied, what helped them "tune in," and why they eventually stopped doing so.

4. Not trying to convince your patients to diet because it's the only way you know to help them with their eating or health problems.

5. If you've dieted, thinking back to how you felt about doing so and how eager you are to restrict calories again.

6. If you've never been a dieter, thinking about the people you've known who have dieted and what it's been like for them.

7. Explaining to patients why diets don't work in the long term.

8. Suggesting that patients read *Secrets from the Eating Lab* by Traci Mann, Ph.D.; *Intuitive Eating* by Evelyn Tribole, M.S., R.D., and Elyse Reich, M.S., R.D.; *Body Respect* by Linda Bacon, Ph.D., and Lucy Aphramor, Ph.D.; and *Health at Every Size* by Linda Bacon, Ph.D.

9. Staying aware of how brainwashed we are about dieting being the answer and slimming down being the solution to virtually every health problem.

Patients, try . . .

1. Being honest about your experiences with dieting—both the hope and the despair you feel or have felt about it.

2. Pledging never to diet again but to take care of your body and health in more effective and sustainable ways.

3. Avoiding engaging in conversations with friends, family, or coworkers about diets or body shaming.

4. Reading books about why diets don't work for the long term, such as *Secrets from the Eating Lab* by Traci Mann, Ph.D.; *Intuitive Eating* by Evelyn Tribole, M.S., R.D., and Elyse Reich, M.S., R.D.; *Body Respect* by Linda Bacon, Ph.D., and Lucy Aphramor, Ph.D.; and *Health at Every Size* by Linda Bacon, Ph.D.

5. Presenting your doctor with a complete diet history whether or not you are asked for one.

6. Not feeling ashamed that diets didn't work for you, even if your health care provider implies that the failure is your fault.

# 4

# Introducing the Dysregulated Eater

## (Hint: You Can't Judge a Book by Its Cover!)

- Ten personality traits of dysregulated eaters
- Co-occurring personality disorders of dysregulated eaters
- Co-occurring mood disorders of dysregulated eaters
- Effects of trauma on dysregulated eating
- Effects of emotional abuse on dysregulated eating

Our hearts go out to doctors and health care providers on the front lines who are dealing with patients' eating and weight concerns (or, sometimes, their apparent *lack* of concern about these issues). In all honesty, you haven't been given many effective tools to work with these difficult problems. It's hard enough for seasoned eating disorder therapists to move clients toward healthier, more appetite-cued eating and taking better care of their bodies. Without addressing the psychological and psychosocial aspects of eating and weight complexities, we believe this challenge is doomed to fail.

We are not trying to turn primary care physicians, nurse practitioners, physicians' assistants, or nurses into Sigmund or Anna Freud. We want only to provide you with the best of what psychology has to offer—information that actually has been available for decades—about how to motivate and work with clients to better manage their food intake and care for their bodies. Nor are we trying to pile on prescriptive lessons atop all the essential things you already do to attend to your job effectively. Based on best practices in the fields of motivation, success, and intuitive eating, our goal is to help you work smarter, not harder.

## THERE'S NO SUCH THING AS YOUR AVERAGE DYSREGULATED EATER WHO STRUGGLES WITH WEIGHT CONCERNS

We all have been taught by this culture to see a heavy person and immediately think that there's something gravely wrong with his or her eating. We also have internalized the corollary that a thin person must be healthy and have nutritional eating habits. Neither assumption is true. We should not assume that a person who wears a size 20 dress or 46 suit doesn't care about health or fitness, or even appearance; that someone who's a svelte six petite must be health conscious; or that average-weight people eat balanced meals and must have an okay relationship with food.

The truth is that we cannot possibly know from a person's size how they eat, what they eat, or how healthy they are. Maybe the thin woman is so obsessed with weight or exercise that she is on a diet that she hates every minute of her life and eats so little that she's not getting enough in the way of nutritious foods. Maybe an average-weight man is engaged in weight cycling, eating non-nutritious (or way too much) food until he gains 10 pounds, then abruptly starving himself until he loses it, over and over again.

The fact is that many people whom we think of as "overweight" would like to be of "normal" weight. For some, this thought may color every waking hour of their lives, but you would never know that to look at them. Sadly, being large in this society may keep their self-esteem low, scare them to death healthwise, restrict their current happiness and charting of future goals, make them fear social intimacy, and cause them to view their size as a deficit no matter how many positive attributes they have going for them. Our point is that providers would do better not making assumptions about weight and eating problems of patients wherever they are on the weight continuum.

## DON'T MOST SERIOUS EATING DISORDERS INVOLVE CALORIC RESTRICTION AND SEVERELY DECREASED FOOD INTAKE?

In terms of mortality, the most serious and deadly of the eating disorders, or as they're called in the DSM-5, "Feeding Disorders," is anorexia nervosa, which is characterized by severe food and caloric restriction in order to attain or maintain a low weight.[1] An equally serious, though less lethal, disorder is bulimia nervosa, which involves binge eating or overeating and subsequent compensatory behaviors, especially purging, to prevent weight gain.[2] New to the DSM-5 as a disorder is binge eating, whose major criterion is frequent episodic ingestion of excessive amounts of food without purging or other compensatory behaviors. Other criteria include ingesting excessive amounts of food in a short period of time, a lack of control over eating, rapid ingestion, feeling uncomfortably full, and experiencing marked distress after eating (ashamed, remorseful, disgusted, self-hating).[3]

Binge eating has long been thought to be rooted in a lack of self-discipline and willpower. Fortunately, recent studies have debunked that myth, including research that "has revealed that high weight in BED is associated with metabolic processes that may exacerbate hunger, prevent satiety, and in some cases, drive food preferences," including the malfunction of hormones such as adipokines, adponectin, gut peptides, and sex hormones.[4] "The cycle of binge eating and weight gain in BED may offer mechanistic insights leading to better treatments not only for BED, but also for obesity in general."[5] What is important about this research, in addition to it pointing to more efficacious treatment directions, is that it takes the stigma off binge eaters and patients of higher weight for being morally inferior due to their excessive food intake.[6]

According to Bunnell and Walsh, Wilfley, and Hudson, the prevalence of binge eating disorder in the community is up to five percent, in weight loss clinics up to 30 percent, and in those with body mass indices (BMI) of 40 or greater, up to 50 percent. According to these prevalence data, in comparison with anorexia or bulimia nervosa, binge eating disorder is the most common eating disorder in existence. Unlike the traditional eating disorders, in binge eating disorder a substantial number of male individuals are affected, with the female to male ratio being 3:2.[7]

Additionally, there is unspecified feeding or eating disorder, which includes disordered eating that does not meet the full criteria for a disorder but causes significant distress and dysfunction in a person's life.[8]

Just because patients do not qualify for a bona fide eating disorder diagnosis, however, does not mean their eating is not severely disordered or, what we would call, dysregulated—mindless, compulsive, or emotional. Another term commonly found in the medical literature is "restrained eating," which means regulating eating by external signals, such as diet rules, rather than with attunement to internal signals of hunger and satiety. According to Linda Bacon, Ph.D., "extensive research suggests that restrained eaters are much less sensitive to hunger and satiety than unrestrained eaters . . . restrained eaters react to emotions and external cues in a nearly totally opposite manner of unrestrained eaters."[9] This point about dysregulated and restrained eaters eating in response to their thoughts and emotions is important to understanding them and why their eating patterns are often as baffling to them as they are to their health care providers. Although these behaviors do not meet a DSM diagnosis, they are as dangerous to patients' physical and mental health as if they did.

The major problem of many patients is that their eating is substantially dysregulated and that they don't feel an internal locus of control over it (which is why they turn to diets for instruction). Some clients might suffer from night eating syndrome, which is awakening and eating in the middle of the night or taking in excessive amounts of food after the dinner hour and before bedtime.[10] The fact is that a great deal of mindless and emotional eating occurs in the hours between dinner time and bed time because this is when patients are bored, lonely, unhappy, looking to de-stress, or simply have gotten into the habit of munching on typical snack foods while watching TV or using the computer. For more information on emotions and eating, we refer you to *The Food & Feelings Workbook* by Karen R. Koenig.

## HOW DO PATIENTS' PERSONALITIES MAKE IT HARDER FOR HEALTH CARE PROVIDERS TO MOVE THEM TOWARD ATTAINING AND MAINTAINING HEALTHY, FUNCTIONAL FOOD AND FITNESS GOALS?

### Personality Traits

When people fail to meet DSM criteria for personality disorders, which you'll learn about later in this chapter, they're said to possess personality traits that cause self- or interpersonal dysfunction. "A personality trait is a tendency to feel, perceive, behave, and think in relatively consistent ways across time and across situations in which the trait may manifest."[11] Obviously, we all have personality traits, not all of which (hopefully) are dysfunctional. The point is that some traits work well for us, such as being reliable or assertive, and some prevent us from having the quality of life we wish to have, such as being unreliable or a pushover.

Traits that make it difficult to eat intuitively, mindfully, and healthfully and engage in physical activity on a consistent basis include (1) categorical (all-or-nothing, black/white and good/bad) thinking, (2) perfectionism, (3) a deficit mindset (focusing on what hasn't been accomplished and has yet to be done rather than on what has been achieved), (4) help avoidance or hyper-responsibility, (5) external rather than internal motivation, (6) people pleasing and approval seeking, (7) a victim mindset, (8) evasion of emotional discomfort, (9) a pattern of acting impulsively, and (10) self-talk about eating, food, fitness, weight, and appearance that is constantly critical, discouraging, punishing, negative, and judgmental.

One overarching characteristic of dysregulated eaters is poor self-care, which occurs on a continuum, from patients who are well put together and look great from the outside to patients whom we recognize are not taking care of themselves the moment they step into our offices. Sure, self-care is about grooming, but it also includes activities such as saying yes and no in the right proportion, carving out alone time, balancing work and play, engaging in effective emotional and stress management, and tending to your needs at least as well and often as you tend to those of others. This kind of self-care is often sorely missing in patients with eating concerns and what gets them into trouble with food. Coincidentally, this is also the kind of care that doctors and medical professionals often lack: while they're taking care of others, who's taking care of them?

If patients don't value themselves or have enough self-esteem to believe they're worth top-notch care and attention, it's going to be an uphill battle to get them to eat well. To mix metaphors, a classic case of putting the cart before the horse. Aside from the aforementioned lack of self-care, here are some dysfunctional personality traits your patients may have.

### Patients who engage in categorical all-or-nothing, black/white, or good/bad thinking

Many people with dysregulated eating engage in mostly all-or-nothing, rigid thinking, not only about food but also in other areas of their lives. They either eat totally nutritiously or go overboard with sugar, fats, and highly processed food. In their minds, foods are labeled as "good" or "bad," with nothing in between, and being good around food feels like a moral imperative to them. They see themselves as successes or failures in eating or exercise (and most of life).

This is why when they eat something "good," they think of themselves as virtuous and proud, and when they eat something "bad," they think of themselves as greedy, disappointing failures.

The terms "good" and "bad" inundate their thoughts, self-talk, and conversations, and, like most people in this culture (maybe even you), they think of eating and exercise in highly moralistic terms. The truth is that a person doesn't don a halo because he or she eats nutritious foods, nor become a bad person because he or she enjoys a steady diet of pizza and Twinkies. This kind of self-judgment is far too simplistic to be mentally healthy or helpful. The words "good" and "bad" are part of diet-speak and the antithesis of the approach that will help our patients. In fact, these words are best avoided completely when referring to health-related behaviors. Stealing, lying, cheating, and harming others are moral issues. Eating a Mars bar is not.

A doctor or health care professional's best strategy in talking with patients with black-and-white thinking is to discuss and emphasize the merits of incremental thinking and learning to enhance long-term behavioral change gradually. It is helpful to speak in terms of progress, baby steps, making consistent efforts, plateaus being necessary resting places, how to get back on track after relapse, being self-compassionate, and the fallibility of humanity. The most useful approach you can take is to praise rigid-thinking patients for their efforts (minimal as they might be) over and over and over again.

### Patients who are perfectionists

Being habituated to perfection is bound to stress out patients (a common trigger for mindless eating) and lead them down the disappointing road to failure one way or another. Either they'll be overwhelmed with unbearable anxiety from struggling to keep up impossibly high standards of eating or exercising or they'll crack under pressure and give up, feeling doomed. This is what the diet mentality has done to us and what we have done to ourselves in our irrational quest for thinness and "good health." Of course, not everyone is perfectionistic, but eating and exercise can be self-destructive paths paved with good intentions in the hands of someone who needs to perform these activities flawlessly in order to have or maintain self-esteem. In fact, one recent study concluded that, compared to women of other weights, "women who are overweight had higher total scores of perfectionism."[12] Moreover, many patients are not only perfectionists around food or fitness. They must do everything (washing dishes, studying for a test, playing tennis, raising their children) so flawlessly that they are stressed when they fail to live up to their excessively high standards and console themselves with food.

Here again, clinicians can play a crucial role in helping patients identify with progress, not perfection. For better or worse, patients may take their cues from their providers. If you're a perfectionist (both authors admittedly have been known to struggle against this tendency), you will want to rein it in when conversing with patients about their eating and fitness goals and avoid placing heavy expectations on them. This is one of those times you will want them to do as you say, not as you might do yourself.

### Patients with a deficit mindset

Patients with dysregulated eating often put far more attention and value on what they haven't accomplished or have yet to achieve than on what they have done well. For a number of reasons, they have difficulty recognizing and acknowledging their strengths and successes and feel unrelenting pressure about all the changes they need to make to "become healthy." In psychotherapy sessions, for example, they will often go on and on about their binges and the times they've engaged in secret or sneak eating and need to be asked if they did *anything* with food or exercise that they considered positive or hopeful recently. Only then will they reveal achievements such as having survived a buffet without overeating, passed up the cookies in the lunch room, hired a trainer, or bought a treadmill. Sadly, their myopia about their achievements needs a cure as much as any other ailments they present with. So, be sure to always ask, "So, tell me, what went well in the self-care department since I saw you last?" You might even start appointments by inquiring about what patients have been doing to take care of themselves, and you will hopefully be surprised by their encouraging baby-step answers.

One caveat: Some patients function in the opposite mode and will tell you only what they did well in the eating or fitness arenas. Too ashamed to reveal their binges or secret overeating or to tell you that they dropped out of the gym a month ago, you may want to praise them to the hills for whatever they've achieved and (this is key) ask, seemingly offhandedly, if there was anything which hasn't been going well or that they regret doing regarding food or fitness. Paradoxically, with these kinds of shame-based patients, you're more likely to hear about backsliding if you act as if it's no big deal and you're only asking to be polite. The more nonjudgmental and compassionate you are, the more they'll cough up where they're having difficulties.

### Patients who are help avoidant

While overly dependent patients might test your forbearance with a panoply of seemingly petty questions that feel urgent to them, there are other patients who will avoid asking for your help about their eating problems at any cost. Most have been brought up to believe they must "be strong" or mustn't burden other people with their problems, and learned early on not to bother soliciting help because it wasn't going to be forthcoming in a caring way. When you sense that they're struggling with food or with staying active and reach out to help these patients, they may act as if everything is fine, there's nothing you can do for them, and they'll handle their problems on their own, thank you very much.

Troubled eaters are highly skilled at covering up their feelings of frustration and despair about ever eating more sanely and healthfully or having the positive body image they desperately wish for. Most live in abject terror of being judged harshly by the world at large and by medical professionals, in particular, so they've learned it's just easier to say they're doing fine—even when their weight gain, blood pressure, or serum cholesterol tell a radically different story. With these clients, the more nonjudgmental and sincere you appear to be in wanting to hear how they're *really* doing, the better the chance that they'll be honest and reach out to you for help. Maybe they'll accept a referral to a dietician, wellness coach, or a therapist. Who knows? You won't have a clue until you ask with kindness, curiosity, empathy, and—above all—compassion. We'll discuss specific how-to strategies in Chapter 7.

### Patients who are externally, rather than internally, motivated

Many troubled eaters are externally motivated to become healthier and that motivation is focused almost entirely on losing weight. We can't blame them. They want to please you as their doctor, to shed pounds for an upcoming wedding or cruise, to have their partner, parent, or children be proud of how they look, and they want their friends to shower them with compliments—and maybe throw a little bit of envy their way as well. Rightly or wrongly, many want to wear current fashions or fit the cultural thin ideal. Their goal might be to reach a specific number on the scale, wear a certain size, or to fit into the tuxedo or dress they wore on their wedding day.

These goals sound commendable until we look at the scientific evidence that says in no uncertain terms that weight loss is *not* the most effective goal for motivating most people to sustain healthy eating behaviors for the long term. Fifty years of psychological research has confirmed repeatedly that in humans, rewards have a complex relationship to motivation. Human nature is such that we do not necessarily internalize motivation based on outcomes or external rewards. In fact, rewards can backfire, so that we are less likely to choose to repeat behaviors that were supported by incentives.[13]

In fact, coaching psychology tells us that the best motivators have been found to be much more personal and tied to values and life vision. For example, a father who travels for work, and thus is faced with heavy restaurant meals every night while on the road, might be more likely to commit to a daily walk or to a salad instead of fries with his meal, because he believes that these behaviors will help him be able to keep up with his children and feel more energetic during family time on weekends. These activities are likely to be much more important to him than seeing a particular number on the scale or BMI chart, although even he may not realize it. That is how motivation works. We and our patients are interested in pretty much the same outcomes: a healthy body, plenty of energy, and zest for life. It's just that patients tend to do better at sustaining the behaviors that promote these outcomes when the behaviors are tied to their values and vision for their best life.

Moreover, nothing tastes or feels better than pride. Interestingly, many troubled eaters are oddly reluctant to use the word pride (one client of Karen's uneasily called it "the P-word" for years), which they associate with boastfulness and excessive self-importance, qualities they were raised to disdain. However, when they understand that pride is nothing more than feeling good about making specific choices that enhance well-being, they begin to comprehend how to grow self-esteem and feel better about valuing taking care of themselves. Even more interestingly, many dysregulated eaters live for others to be proud of them but shrug off being proud of themselves. This externally oriented dynamic, in a nutshell (and explained in more detail below), helps us understand why so many of them fail at sustaining healthy behaviors.

### Patients who are people pleasers and approval seekers

One kind of external motivation in particular stands out and is highly relevant to this book: the desire to please others, especially authority figures, in this case *you*, a doctor, or other health care professional. At first glance, this may seem like a win-win situation: your patient brings in the great news that he or she is starting to eat more normally and nutritiously and gives you the credit for making it happen, perhaps starting the conversation by saying, "You're going to be so proud of me." You smile and can't help but feel encouraged. Your patient feels great and so do you.

But with further scrutiny, do you really want your patients to be doing things for *you* to be proud of *them* or do you want your patients to enhance their health so that *they* will be proud of *themselves*? Be careful of this trap. When patients openly seek your approval, they are taking the exact wrong route to success.[14] Sure, you can feel happy for them and their achievements, but *they* must be the ones to feel proud of their achievements because that's the only thing that matters and is going to keep them consistently chugging along to do more of the same in the future—unless you're willing to be intimately involved in their daily lives, cheering them along, for the rest of your time on earth.

The idea is to encourage patients to approve of and be proud of themselves. Wanting to please you or anyone else may get them started on the right track, but it's not going to keep them going. For that, they will need a locus of motivation within them: to own their achievements, be their best cheerleader, and take time and mindful space to celebrate small successes (even for a brief moment, giving themselves an internal "good for me!"). When they speak of you being proud of them, you can sidestep the tribute and help them enormously by saying, "What matters is that you learn to be proud of yourself."

### Patients who view themselves as victims

Many health care professionals find it difficult if not impossible to help people who have a victim mentality: these poor souls live under a dark cloud, don't have any luck except bad luck, never catch a break, have a million and one excuses about why they can't eat better or become more active, and don't want to even bother trying to get healthy because they've tried before and it hasn't worked, don't ya know? Sometimes they act as if not one good thing ever has happened in their whole lives and they aren't expecting their fortune to turn around just because of a few appointments with you.

Patients with a victim mindset can be a big challenge. You try to motivate them until they "yes-but" you to death so that you throw up your metaphoric hands in frustration. The truth is that in your brief time with them, you're not going to suddenly reverse years or, more likely decades, of their feeling like the underdog or last week's garbage. Perhaps the most you can do is to find a therapist who will support them in exploring their beliefs about their powerlessness. Your best bet in this situation is to keep your compassion high and your referral list of skilled therapists close at hand.

### Patients who evade emotional discomfort

Few people joyously seek out emotional discomfort or psychic dissonance, but there are some folks who are champions at avoiding it at all costs. At the slightest flicker of emotional distress, they distract themselves. Psychotherapists call this duck-and-cover reaction Experiential Avoidance (EA), which "is a coping style characterized by the tendency to try to change or get rid of unwanted thoughts, feelings or bodily sensations. EA can be harmful because a rigid focus on short-term relief or comfort can sometimes come at the expense of long-term functioning."[15] Patients engaging in EA will seek out food or any kind of momentary distraction. They don't actually get to avoid distress, however; they only exchange whatever uncomfortable feeling they're experiencing *before* eating with a battery of painful emotions *after* mindless eating such as guilt, shame, remorse, self-hate, despair, and so forth.

What you experience with them as patients in your office is this same kind of EA reaction. You raise an uncomfortable subject (their bad knees, hypertension, high cholesterol, diabetes, etc.) and they become so distressed that they change topics or execute some other communication maneuver to feel better. It's fine to bring them back to the topic at hand, as long as you understand that their modus operandi is nothing personal.

These individuals either don't understand how short-term emotional discomfort leads to long-term life enhancement or lack the skills to tolerate unpleasant feelings even if they wanted to bear them. While your impulse, in this case, may be to ramp up their discomfort (in case they missed your point the first two times you brought it up), this tactic is doomed to failure and will only make them more well defended. Instead, drop the subject and try again another time. It's fine to say something such as "The subject of eating and health is often hard for my patients to talk about. In my experience, it can stir up a lot of uncomfortable feelings."

### Patients who often act impulsively

Taking care of our health effectively involves a great deal of foresight, planning, and monitoring, including planning meals, reading nutritional labels, keeping a stocked pantry, and, of course, cooking. Even restaurant meals take some planning: where to go and what to eat. It also takes deliberate intent to get exercise on a regular basis. We need to make time for it, ensure that it's a priority, and fit it into our busy schedules. When patients are generally impulsive, especially if self-care is not a priority for them, they often have a difficult time doing relatively simple tasks consistently. Moreover, if they cannot easily tolerate frustration or defer gratification, it will be a source of misery for them to keep to a routine with food or regular exercise. These are your patients who "forget" to take their medications daily or even brush their teeth.

Those of us who have a fairly high frustration tolerance and are relatively easily able to delay gratification (like those in the medical field who spent a fortune and many years of arduous work getting to where they are now) might find it mind-boggling that patients can make the erratic decisions they do and fail so utterly to plan ahead when it's obvious that they need to. It's not unusual for impulsive people to clear all the "junk" food out of their house in the morning in one fell swoop, then pass by the supermarket in the afternoon and restock their pantry with these same exact items. Such seemingly "self-sabotaging" moves are often indicators of mixed feelings or internal conflict, or even of an ongoing reaction to a deprivation mindset caused or exacerbated by years of chronic dieting. We will discuss this situation in more detail in Chapter 5. These actions are more about gratification (short-term pleasure) than about happiness (long-term pleasure), and many patients don't realize that sometimes they can't have both.

With patients who are impulsive, you, as a health care provider, cannot expect miracles and will need to markedly lower your expectations of what they can achieve and how fast they can achieve it. It is not your job to teach your patients how to think and act rationally. Nor is it within the scope of your duties to provide patients with a crash course on effective decision-making and goal setting. If you suspect that they have attention and impulsivity problems that strongly affect their functioning and self-care, you may want to enlist the aid of a psychotherapist to help them learn new skills so that you can work with them more effectively.

**Patients whose self-talk about eating, food, fitness, weight, and appearance is constantly critical, discouraging, negative, punishing, and judgmental**

If we are, in large part, what we think we are, then, to succeed, we need to have positive thoughts about who we are and what we are doing. However, this is exactly the opposite of the self-talk of many people who have eating and weight concerns. They regularly compare themselves to others and fail to measure up. They are immensely hard on themselves for their weight and their "out of control" eating (and many other activities). Their constant mind chatter is full of self-shaming, self-loathing, and condemnation. No matter what their accomplishments, they end up focusing on their failures. All that matters, they tell themselves, is that they *are* fat, *feel* fat, *hate* fat, and will probably always *be* fat.

They are generally people who have enormous compassion for others (including you, their provider, who they believe is stuck treating them) and next to nothing for themselves. The negative chatter running through their head must be turned off and tuned out if they are to make progress on the health front. Only when self-talk reverses itself from negative and critical to positive and compassionate will patients change their behavior on a consistent basis.

One of the best ways to help patients stop the negative blah, blah, blah is to show deep empathy and compassion for them. Shaming them only makes them feel more worthless and shame, rather than motivating them, actually does the opposite and causes them to feel as if they are right to not value themselves. What a negative spiral this produces. And what a positive spiral you can generate from the simple, human act of showing compassion to patients, whatever size they are.

---

Brain food for providers: Thinking about the patients you see regularly, can you identify any of the above personality traits in them? What could you do to have more compassion for and work better with them?

---

Brain food for patients: Do you have any of the above traits? What would you like your health care providers to know about you that would make your relationship work better, especially when talking about your health? How would you like to modify your traits to work better with your providers or enhance your chances of success?

## WHAT ABOUT DYSREGULATED EATERS WHO HAVE
## MORE MARKED PERSONALITY DYSFUNCTION?

Psychology differentiates between personality disorders and personality traits and some of your patients may have underlying disorders. According to the DSM-5™, "A personality disorder is an enduring pattern of inner experience and behavior that deviates markedly from the expectations of the individual's culture, is pervasive and inflexible, has an onset in adolescence or early adulthood, is stable over time, and leads to distress or impairment" in functioning.[16]

You don't need to be a psychotherapist to recognize if a patient has a personality disorder. You just need to consider the possibility and have a general idea of the criteria for the most likely ones you'll encounter. We know them when we see them or, more accurately, when we interact with an individual who has one. You might think of personality-disordered folks as difficult people who have a pattern of being rude or rebellious, calling you excessively about minor issues, expecting special treatment, lying about or refusing to discuss their health problems, needing to be dragged into your office by loved ones or dragged out once you get them talking, constantly running off on tangents, rebelliously viewing you as the enemy, or acting as if they were powerless victims incapable of improving the quality of their lives.

### Co-occurring Personality Disorders

Personality can play several major roles for those with eating disorders: as a risk factor, as a moderator of symptomatic expression, in choice of treatment, and also as a predictive factor in outcome. Some personality traits are common to all eating disorders, while others are strongly related only to certain types of eating disorders, such as high perfectionism in anorexia nervosa (AN) and increased sensation-seeking in binge eating disorder.[17]

Several types of personality disorders may make it difficult for patients to take care of their health effectively by engaging in activities such as in nutrition-minded grocery shopping, planning ahead (an oddly difficult task for many dysfunctional eaters who are otherwise quite functional) and preparing healthy meals, eating mindfully, and getting or staying in shape. In truth, some patients are able to *do* all of the above activities, but generally not consistently or for long. We're not expecting you to learn to assign a mental health diagnosis to all of your patients. Rather, we're hoping that when you spot a particular trait or disorder, it will click in your mind why your patient might be having a hard time listening to you or taking your advice about health and wellness, and that you will respond with compassion and caring.

Below are brief descriptions of the personality disorders you may encounter with your patients who have eating and weight concerns, with the important caveat that, of course, not all patients with dysregulated eating or weight concerns have any of them.

Borderline Personality Disorder (BPD) "is a pattern of instability in interpersonal relationships, self-image, and affects, and marked impulsivity."[18] Patients with this disorder may:

- Have unstable relationships, putting you up on a pedestal for several appointments, treating you as a god and insisting that you're the best doctor in the world, and then showing up at another appointment furious that you suggested they might benefit from an antidepressant to help reduce their anxiety, which causes them to binge, or see a psychotherapist to help with their impulsivity or low self-esteem.
- Give you double messages that make you feel both sorry for them as victims (as they often see themselves) and also makes you angry at them if they lash out at you.
- Have great difficulty with emotional regulation, especially self-soothing (there is a high correlation between BPD and bulimia and binge eating disorder).
- Seem to push a great many of your buttons (or those of your staff), though you're not sure why.
- Seem oversensitive and cause you to feel you need to walk on eggshells around them.
- Be manipulative and lie about their weight or what they're eating, although inside they are frightened, fragile people living in a high-stress world with few comfort or coping skills.
- Have an unstable sense of self, which is characterized by experiencing a sudden drop or escalation in perception of self-worth based on external factors—a compliment or insult, praise or criticism, rejection/abandonment/ betrayal, or success or failure in achieving a goal.
- Easily become emotionally triggered by internal cues—a favorable or unfavorable comparison of self to another, the trigger of memories of feeling

undervalued or unloved, self-judgment of poor decision-making, or a reaction to the number on the scale traveling up or down.

"Up to 53.8% of patients with borderline personality disorder also meet criteria for an eating disorder, and up to 21.7% of patients with borderline personality disorder meet criteria specifically for anorexia nervosa and 24.1%, specifically for bulimia nervosa."[19] BPD can be characterized by "impulsive and often dangerous behaviors, such as spending sprees, unsafe sex, substance abuse, reckless driving, and *binge eating*" (italics ours).[20] Research on personality and eating styles even suggests that "neurotic and emotionally unstable individuals seem to adopt counter-regulatory external or emotional eating and eat high-energy dense sweet and savory foods."[21]

Helping patients with BPD get into therapy if they aren't already engaged in it may be the best approach health care providers can take, while putting aside discussions on eating and weight concerns until the patient is more stable, less impulsive, and more trusting of a provider. Consistently letting these patients know you care about them and walking the fine line between not being put off by their sometimes difficult personalities and setting limits for them in your office may be the wisest effort you can make on their (and your) behalf.

Avoidant Personality Disorder (APD) "is a pattern of social inhibition, feelings of inadequacy, and hypersensitivity to negative evaluation."[22] Patients with this disorder may:

- See negative judgment in practically every suggestion you make, no matter how benign your words are, how kind your tone is, or how helpful your intent is.
- Be especially sensitive to fat stigma and may feel a great deal of shame (perhaps even more than you can imagine) about their bodies.
- Talk about absolutely anything but what you wish to discuss about their eating or weight.
- Keep changing the subject, go off on wild tangents, bombard you with questions to avoid delving into a distressing topic, or fail to keep appointments when they haven't done what you've asked or what they promised they'd do.

Really, they're not avoiding you; they're avoiding their internal distress and problems. If you two were discussing your favorite movies, they'd probably love to stay and chat. Feel free to patiently and tactfully bring them back to the health topic at hand or give it another try at another appointment.

Dependent Personality Disorder (DPD) "is a pervasive and excessive need to be taken care of that leads to submissive and clingy behavior and fears of separation."[23] Patients with this disorder may:

- Require frequent reminders about what actions to take and wish to put you in the position of being responsible for their success in taking care of their health.
- Have tremendous anxiety about making decisions and being or doing wrong.
- Need a great deal of advice and reassurance from health care providers that they're doing the best thing or doing it well enough.
- Need far more support and reassurance than you can possibly give them.
- Have great difficulty being accountable for what they promise to do between appointments and for being responsible for themselves.
- Feel shame and self-contempt for their perceived ineptitude and ineffectiveness, and especially for their dependence on others.

If patients with APD can't wait to leave your office, those with DPD would be happy to have you on call 24/7 to help them and tell them what to do. Many of them act helpless (consciously or unconsciously) in order to have caring people in their lives, believing that if they succeed, they will be abandoned and, therefore, alone. Be patient and compassionate, and you will earn their trust, especially if you approach them in a collaborative style.

### HOW DO MOOD DISORDERS AFFECT TREATMENT OF PATIENTS WITH DYSREGULATED EATING OR WEIGHT DISSATISFACTION?

The answer, in a word, is that mood disorders have a huge impact on the origins and treatment of eating and weight concerns, far more than most health care providers might expect. Patients who have Generalized Anxiety Disorder (GAD) or who are easily stressed might be inclined to de-stress by heading for a carbohydrate fix more than patients who are not particularly anxiety prone in the first place. It is the constancy and the intensity of GAD coupled with the accessibility of food that makes refraining from mindless eating so arduous. Just as saying "eat less" doesn't do the trick because many patients don't have the skills to do so, saying "be less anxious" works just as poorly.

Patients who have depressive disorders may feel equally powerless to improve their eating or fitness, and their low energy level and lethargy will make it difficult for them to get out and exercise or, perhaps, even go grocery shopping. Moreover, their despair may cause them to feel that it doesn't matter if they eat "junk food" because they may believe they'll never reach their goals or that they don't deserve to live a healthy life. We've all been around long enough to know that depression can undermine self-care, even if patients have the best intentions when they are in your office.

Moreover, "A new study in the *Journal of the Academy of Nutrition and Dietetics (JAND)* points to obesity and depression as co-conspirators undermining the health of people in low-income neighborhoods characterized as food deserts." Researchers found that "higher scores on depression predicted both higher BMI and lower dietary quality. And then there is the understanding that adverse childhood experiences are an important risk factor for depression, as well as it is for obesity. These experiences paint an increasingly clear picture about why simplistic efforts to urge people to move more and eat better are not moving the needle on obesity in these communities."[24]

Patients who carry a diagnosis of Bipolar Disorder may be gung ho to follow healthful routines when they are in the manic or hypomanic phase of their disorder. However, as their mood plummets and they begin the gradual (or, for rapid-cyclers, swift) descent into depression, they may grab fast food every day because they're too fatigued to food shop, and keep their running shoes and water bottle by the front door, but never use them.

## HOW DOES HAVING POSTTRAUMATIC STRESS DISORDER (PTSD) AFFECT EATING PROBLEMS?

There is no one way that PTSD will affect patients with eating and weight concerns. Depending on the stresses in their lives, especially triggering situations, they may have different reactions. They may suffer from depression and may have limited energy for or interest in taking care of themselves. They might be passive and overly compliant because they fear you'll be angry with them if they don't do exactly as you say, or they may be aggressive and belligerent due to anger management issues. Some truly may have difficulty with concentration and may not be able to follow an eating plan or activity schedule because their thoughts are preoccupied with ensuring that they feel safe. Moreover, it's important to remember that witnessing violence or a horrific event can be as traumatic for patients as having experienced the event themselves.

About one-quarter of people who binge eat have PTSD. "People with PTSD have such a hard time focusing on the present and future because they are preoccupied with traumatic memories or trying to avoid traumatic reminders," says Rachel Yehuda, Ph.D., director of the traumatic stress studies division at the Icahn School of Medicine at Mount Sinai in New York. "Sometimes that means they don't plan well for future meals, and [as a result], they may get very hungry and overeat or overeat compulsively."[25]

Of course, there is no reason you would know any of this unless you are aware of their diagnosis. If you suspect a patient has PTSD, you might try gently bringing up the subject and see where that gets you. If patients have been treated for trauma in psychotherapy, they will likely be more willing to talk about it than if they've been keeping it a secret for months, years, or decades.

## ARE THERE OTHER MENTAL HEALTH ISSUES THAT COULD POTENTIALLY PREVENT PATIENTS FROM RESOLVING EATING PROBLEMS AND TAKING BETTER CARE OF THEIR HEALTH?

You might already know that there is a high correlation between trauma (even in the absence of PTSD) and eating disorders. Because binge eating disorder has only recently been added to the DSM-5 as a stand-alone, bona fide diagnosis, it is less likely to be associated with trauma than anorexia or bulimia nervosa. Even chronic overeating or unhealthy eating may have subclinical correlations to trauma and we simply do not have the research to prove it yet.

Timberline Knolls, a residential eating disorder treatment center, says this about trauma, its nuances, and its repercussions:

Trauma is defined as any injury, whether physically or emotionally inflicted. In psychiatry, trauma refers to an overwhelming experience that is physically and emotionally painful, distressful, or shocking, which often results in lasting effects. In the behavioral health field, trauma is separated into two categories: discrete traumas (sometimes called big "T" trauma) and chronic, insidious traumas (sometimes called little "t" trauma). Basically, these categories are predicated on frequency and severity.

Discrete trauma is a highly identifiable and catastrophic event, including severe physical abuse, rape, extreme injury, witnessing violence, or an unexpected death of a relative or friend. Vivid and explicit memories usually, but not always, surround this type of trauma. Chronic trauma is less about one identifiable event and more about reoccurring painful situations or experiences, such as ongoing parental criticism, childhood neglect, being bullied or teased, or experiencing alcoholism, another addiction or mental/medical illness in the family. The ongoing nature and the more "acceptable" aspect of this type of emotional trauma often makes it more difficult to identify and treat.[26]

Note that being bullied or teased is exactly what many high-weight patients have experienced, sometimes since childhood.

"There is a strong correlation between trauma and eating disorders. A number of studies have shown that people who struggle with eating disorders have a higher incidence of neglect and physical, emotional and sexual abuse. In particular, binge eating disorder is associated with emotional abuse while sexual abuse has been linked to eating disorders in males. An eating disorder may develop in an attempt to cope with the trauma, suppress painful emotions or to regain a sense of control. Individuals with a history of trauma may not fully recover from an eating disorder, or may experience chronic relapse from their eating disorder until they address the underlying trauma." Moreover, and vital for health care providers to remember, "A traumatic experience in childhood can manifest as an eating disorder years later."[27]

Numerous studies have looked at how trauma may be a causative factor in obesity. For example, "In a study of 286 obese people in the program," Vincent J. Felitti, M.D., coprincipal investigator of the Adverse Childhood Experiences (ACE) Study, doing ongoing collaborative research between the Kaiser Permanente Medical Care Program and the Centers for Disease Control, "discovered that half had been sexually abused as children. For these people, overeating and obesity weren't the central problems, but attempted solutions. Food was an old, reliable friend that soothed and calmed them, while being fat protected them from a hostile world."[28]

The article goes on to say, "Notwithstanding all the bean counters obsessing about cost containment, the vast implications of this study—medical, social, political—seem to trigger a kind of cognitive dissonance in the world of health care. The medical profession isn't designed, organized, or financed, much less philosophically ready, to grapple with these facts. Rather than exploring amorphous, hard-to-measure psychosocial and emotional factors lost in the mists of time and patients' unverifiable memories, both medical researchers and clinicians focus on what's directly in front of them—current physical symptoms and directly preceding causes. So the traumatic 'insults' in childhood to complex neurobiological systems remain 'silent' until the middle-aged or elderly patient brings her obesity and diabetes, his high blood pressure and clogged arteries, to a physician half a century or more later."[29]

This is particularly true of childhood or adolescent sexual abuse. According to the National Eating Disorders Association, "Particularly with child sexual abuse (CSA), there has been a large amount of research related to the effect of CSA on body image. It is believed that 30% of individuals with an eating disorder have been sexually abused. Some researchers connect the large association of self-harm with victims of CSA and other traumas to those with eating disorders. Those at high risk for eating disorders because of trauma include: victims of sexual abuse, particularly those who suffered at a younger age, and victims or observers of domestic violence."[30]

"Scientists don't yet know exactly how PTSD and binge eating are linked in the body. Both conditions are related to problems with stress hormones and mood-boosting brain chemicals, though, research shows. Your genes might also determine whether or not you get these two disorders.[31] More often than not, the trauma (which leads to PTSD) comes first and the binge eating comes later. Scientists think people binge eat to 'escape' the painful memories related to the traumatic event. 'People with Binge Eating Disorder often don't understand what they're feeling or why,' says Timothy Brewerton, MD, executive medical director of The Hearth Center for Eating Disorders in Columbia, S.C. 'They're too busy compulsively trying to numb the pain with food.'"[32]

Most of the time, patients who are trauma survivors and have eating and weight concerns won't necessarily put two and two together when talking with health care providers. They won't say, "I was sexually abused by my stepfather for three years and now I am more comfortable being fat than being thin because I feel that somehow my size protects me from being sexually assaulted" or "When my gym teacher sexually abused me after soccer practice, I would always go home and raid the refrigerator to numb out my feelings."

## DOES A PATIENT HAVING BEEN ABUSED RISE TO THE LEVEL OF TRAUMA?

Emotional abuse may have a strong, serious and long-standing effect on a person, yet not reach the level of big T trauma. Verbal and emotional abuse, especially shaming, can have a lasting impact on one's eating and self-image. One study exploring the role of childhood emotional abuse (CEA) as a predictor of disordered eating found that "CEA had a direct, unmediated effect on eating pathology."[33]

Here are several kinds of behaviors that occur in childhood which, if they happen on a regular basis, have a lasting negative effect on self-image, identity, and general functionality—and often, eating. Although you and they may not recognize the impact of such behaviors on your patients' ability to engage in positive self-care, invalidation, shaming, humiliation, and bullying have a strong negative effect on developing self-esteem.

### Invalidation

Invalidation causes children to disconnect from feelings and sensations, assuming they are wrong or bad. For example, when Mom asks (which sounds more like telling) the child, "You're not *really* angry, are you?" the child may think, "I guess I shouldn't be angry, that I'm a bad person for being angry that Mom forgot to pick me up after debate club today." Or the child may feel invalidated if he's still hungry after his plate is taken away before he's finished eating, and think to himself, "Dad said he doesn't want me to get fat and took away my plate, so I must be full."

Lack of self-trust in one's feelings due to emotional invalidation is a major issue for dysregulated eaters. They often lack the ability to identify what they think or feel, are filled with self-doubt and self-mistrust, and are constantly second-guessing themselves. They actually can be unsure if they are hungry, full, satisfied, or have eaten enough, because they've disconnected from their internal cues for eating, and in other ways as well. They regularly confuse affect sensation for hunger and may routinely eat in a misguided attempt to comfort themselves when they are bored, lonely, sad, anxious, or even tired. It's easy to appreciate how such behaviors and habits could ultimately manifest as an uncomfortably high or steadily increasing weight for such patients, despite their "trying to eat better." Importantly, these patients are often completely unaware of the emotional and self-regulatory skill sets that they lack. Maintaining a high index of suspicion regarding the possibility of an inadequate emotional regulation skill set can increase your effectiveness in serving and supporting these patients immeasurably. A sensitive question or timely referral to a therapist or qualified coach can be the first step toward healing and improvement in self-efficacy.

### Shaming

A major kind of abuse, which may be traumatizing, is when children are shamed for their bodies or eating behaviors, whether by parents, relatives, adults they know, strangers, or other children. When shame and eating pathology is studied, "findings revealed the impact of shame memories on eating psychopathology is completely moderated by social comparisons based on physical appearance. These results showcase the significance of early shame experiences including peers and other social agents that become traumatic memories, central to self-identity, to eating disorder patients' perceptions of inferiority and their core psychopathology features."[34]

There is no way for you to know about these experiences unless you ask about previous trauma or shaming, but, even then, patients may not tell you because they may feel responsible for what occurred (e.g., for being abused or assaulted) and, therefore, deeply ashamed. Alternately, they may not want to trigger their own distress by talking about it. Dysregulated eating is a shame-based behavior and may often come from growing up in a shame-based household. Once again, your empathy, compassion, and sensitive inquiry can be a corrective, healing experience.

### Humiliation and Bullying

One more type of trauma is relevant to this discussion—the shame of being humiliated or bullied because of one's weight. Some patients have suffered terribly in childhood, adolescence, and adulthood for being a higher than average weight. They have been physically hurt, excluded from activities, laughed at and made fun of, and can barely think or talk about their eating or weight without tail-spinning back into memories of these horrors. We, as health care providers, would do well to remember that this experience with weight stigma has the potential to cause much more long-term damage than the presence of extra fat.

It is your recognition that these patients have suffered from bullying which will help you be compassionate with them. And it is your caring and compassion which can help them look at how their suffering affects their eating and seek treatment so that they can truly put it behind them.

In summary, in the brief time allotted to you—perhaps over the long haul—it pays for you to get to know your patients with eating and weight concerns inside out. Maybe it's by asking a routine question about their relationship with food and if they're happy or unhappy with their health. Maybe it's by adding a few questions about eating or perceived weight stigma on your medical intake form in the social history section. Each one of your patients with eating and weight concerns is uniquely more than meets the eye and has an individual story behind how he or she arrived at having a poor or unsatisfying relationship with food and body image. The more you know and understand about this relationship, the more effective a clinician you'll be and the more these patients will value and heal from your help.

---

Brain food for providers: How have mood or personality disorders or having suffered trauma affected your discussions with patients about treatment of their eating and weight concerns? What would you like to do differently in the future to improve their treatment?

---

Brain food for patients: How have mood disorders or having experienced trauma, weight stigma, or abuse affected your relationship with food and your body? What would you like your providers to know about these issues and how to treat you?

---

Providers, try . . .

1. Recognizing that each patient has a unique combination of physical traits, medical conditions, diet history, genetic temperament, personality traits, and mental health issues that will make it easier or harder for him or her to eat "normally" and healthfully consistently and become and remain fit.
2. Getting to know the eating disorders therapists in your community, or contacting your nearest eating disorders treatment center for names of outpatient clinicians or coaches who work with emotional and binge eating.
3. Asking open-ended questions about whether patients have depression and anxiety problems or have suffered trauma or abuse, explaining how all of these can affect weight and dysregulate affect and eating.
4. Leading with caring, compassion, and empathy when talking to trauma survivors with eating and weight concerns.
5. Reacting without judgment, no matter what patients tell you in the area of eating and weight.

6. When necessary, making the case for psychotherapy for patients who have been struggling for a long time or are frustrated with their lack of progress in managing their eating problems.
7. Treating patients the way you wish your family members or friends with mental health issues would be treated in medical settings.

Patients, try . . .

1. Having positive expectations of medical visits and giving yourself time to get to know a practitioner and for him or her to get to know you.
2. Not being defensive when asked a question about food or weight and answering honestly.
3. Reflecting upon your feelings as a patient struggling with eating and weight concerns, and whether you might benefit from support from a psychotherapist, lifestyle medicine practitioner, dietician, coach, trainer, or a group focused on enhancing life skills for a better relationship with food and your body.
4. Telling providers what they do well and could do better regarding your eating and weight concerns.
5. Being curious and not defensive if your provider suggests that you might be suffering from depression, anxiety, or some other mental health problem.
6. Reading up on how trauma, neglect, abuse, depression, and anxiety can trigger and adversely impact dysregulated eating.
7. Being honest and open with your providers about your eating habits, even secret eating, hoarding food, binge eating, purging, extreme food restriction, or taking laxatives.

# 5

# How Dysregulated Eaters Become "Normal" Eaters

## (It's about Self-care, Not Just Health Care!)

- Helping dysregulated eaters have a better relationship with food and improved body image
- How poor self-care, irrational beliefs, mixed feelings, and inadequate life skills underlie dysregulated eating
- Guidelines for "normal" eating
- The difference between "normal" and nutritious eating

Hopefully, by now, you're starting to understand that dysregulated eaters have underlying challenges that affect their eating, self-care, and health. Later in this chapter, we will tell you how to help them improve their relationship with food and their bodies and become "normal" eaters, but, for now, it's important to learn a bit more about the dysregulated eaters you see in your practice. There is much more to know than meets the eye.

How can you recognize which of your patients are dysregulated eaters? Obviously, some of them may raise their eating or health concerns when they first meet you. Or you may meet a patient and, because of his or her large size, bring up the subjects of eating and exercise. Other patients may have a low or average weight, yet have dysregulated eating that you are unaware of. They may be caught up in the diet-binge cycle and simply believe that's how they'll live out their whole lives. They may be average size or slim, but eat in a way that does not contribute to health or longevity. Or they may "watch their weight" so closely that, though obsessed by food and weight, they never allow themselves to gain a pound. These are all forms of dysregulated eating.

Just as you can't judge a book by its cover, you can't assess health by looking at someone's size or weight. It may surprise you to learn that many patients who are highly successful, functional, and well put together live in daily distress over food. They're so ashamed of their eating behaviors that they wouldn't dare tell you about them. They figure that if they look good from the outside, no one will ever know how badly they're doing (with food and life) on the inside.

One approach is to ask patients how their relationship with food is. If you notice blood pressure, cholesterol, and triglyceride numbers which are not within a healthy range, feel free to ask with a neutral, not a condemnatory, tone, "How do you feel about your eating?" or "What's your relationship with food like?" and wait to see what answer you receive. Another avenue is to build a nonjudgmental, caring relationship with them so that they begin to trust you enough to see that you want to help them. Make no assumptions, use active listening skills, ask open-ended questions, and look for conversational openings when they may make references to any kind of eating concerns. Remember, the more together patients appear, the harder it may be for them to disclose eating difficulties.

## I'M NO SHRINK, SO ONCE I IDENTIFY DYSREGULATED EATERS IN MY PRACTICE, HOW DO I HELP THEM IMPROVE THEIR RELATIONSHIP WITH FOOD AND THEIR BODIES?

In graduate school, it is pounded into the heads of social work students to view the client in context and to think in psychosocial terms. Their view is the panorama of a client's life, going deeply into their histories and spreading outward into the present. It is also recommended for doctors treating patients with eating and weight concerns to take this broader view as well.[1]

From the psychosocial viewpoint, every factor is fair game when assessing what is happening with a client. Using this perspective, it is useful to consider: (1) how clients *take care of themselves* in general (which is based, in large part, on how their parents or caretakers took care of them), (2) what they *believe* about food, eating, weight, and appearance as well as the core beliefs they live by that generate self-esteem and self-worth (which develop from what their culture and family believed and how they were treated), (3) how well or poorly they *manage life* (which skills were or weren't modeled and taught by family and gained through outside experiences), and (4) how they are able to resolve any *mixed feelings* about eating and weight issues (also derived from family and culture).

In this chapter, we'll explore and address some of the more subtle and often invisible but powerful ways that psychosocial factors affect the patients we meet in our medical offices every day. First, we'll look at what could cause people to develop an unhealthy relationship with food and their bodies; then we'll explain what "normal" and nutritious eating are, how they differ, and ways in which you can guide dysregulated eaters to have a sane, healthy relationship with food and their bodies.

Please don't take it personally and get angry at your patients for failing to do what they said they'd do: start that walking program they swore they'd begin last year or follow the food plan their diabetes educator gave them. However poorly your patient is doing, it's the best he or she can do at that moment. Remember, hard as it may be to accept, we all are doing the best we can in any given moment based on our histories, circumstances, and internal resources—even though how or what we're doing may not be good enough. Accepting this axiom may seem contrary to common sense because it makes us feel as if we're letting folks off the hook and not keeping them accountable, as if we're saying it's okay that they're taking the easy way out. But that's not what we're saying or doing, and the principle makes complete sense when you carefully think it through.

For example, say you run a race as fast as you can, beating all your previous records and most of your competitors, but still come in last. You are doing the best you can, but it's not good enough to win or place in the race. If a therapist follows every clinical guideline to save a client from committing suicide and the client does it anyway, the therapist has done the best he could, but it wasn't enough to prevent a client's death by his own hand. If a surgeon performs a successful kidney transplant, but the patient develops a rejection reaction, the surgeon has done the best she could, but it was still not good enough to ensure an optimal outcome.

The idea is that we all are functioning at our highest level every moment of our lives based on factors too numerous and complex to discuss here. For many people—and many patients—their best is woefully deficient and inadequate. Not everyone's best is good or even approaches mediocre. Some of us will do better than others simply by virtue of the fact that we all don't start off on a level playing field. The bright note in this sobering admission is that people can learn new skills and do often improve, so that their best becomes better and eventually good enough.

So, let's assume that your patients with eating and weight concerns are doing the best they can around food, which currently might be poorly. With help, terrible self-care may rise to middling, and fair self-care may rise to good. It's no use being angry at patients for taking poor or even downright awful care of themselves—eating a constant diet of high-sugar and highly processed foods, being a total couch potato, not taking their medicine, failing to follow through on the testing you repeatedly and urgently recommend with the noblest of intentions. Most can—and will—improve with the right guidance. What they often need are some learnable self-care and life skills.

Here are some ideas to consider when patients are not doing as well at improving their health as you and they had hoped.

### Self-care

There are numerous reasons that people don't take good care of themselves consistently. Some had substandard role models in their parents or grew up in conditions of poverty, wretchedness, or crime-ridden neighborhoods in which food was scarce and self-care was narrowly defined as not getting yourself killed. Maybe your patients' families had no health insurance or had distressing or disastrous experiences at hospitals or neighborhood clinics. Many of your patients—no matter how self-assured and accomplished they may appear!—may have been mistreated emotionally, sexually, or physically as children and, deep down, don't believe they deserve to take care of their bodies or their minds. If your patients grew up lounging in front of the TV snarfing down Doritos or canned spaghetti for dinner every night while their parents were minding their other children, out working, or even in another room getting drunk, they never may have actually been well cared for and may be clueless as adults about what caring for oneself physically or emotionally entails.

Patients may have had their eating in childhood inappropriately micromanaged or neglected entirely. They may have been of "normal weight" but their parents feared them getting fat (because it ran in the family) and supervised every morsel that went into their children's mouths. Some were raised in families where emotions were aired too publicly and uncontrollably or where feelings were never expressed, so that they never learned effective emotional management skills, which puts them at high risk for emotional eating. It is vitally important not to make any assumptions about patients' eating because they seem to be living the good life. Often it's these patients, whose lives look so good on the outside, who feel like a mess on the inside and end up struggling with food.

In order to take good care of ourselves, we need to have had caretakers who more often than not adequately met our mental, emotional, and physical needs, so we could then internalize doing this for ourselves. We cannot stress strongly enough that many people—many of your patients—have poor self-care because they were never taught to care for themselves. For many, being poorly cared for left them (perhaps unconsciously) believing they weren't worth the trouble; hence, they don't value themselves enough to take the trouble now. Even for those who were well cared for in childhood, repeated cycles of restrictive dieting, deprivation, and "failure" to attain a comfortable weight may have undermined these patients' positive body image, self-efficacy, and feelings of self-worth, leaving them fluctuating between self-care and "I don't care."

Sadly, they may view your efforts in caring for them as a waste of time or themselves as a lost cause. Though it might be hard to believe, you may be the first person in a very long time who has taken a real interest in how they are faring in this area. Therefore, it may take a while for your caring to sink in.

Treating patients who have internalized worthlessness can be a one-step-forward-and-two-steps-backward affair. You finally get them to monitor their diabetes daily and they slack off taking walks with the "Sunday morning walkers" club they joined. Or you manage to call in a favor to slip them into a stress management group, and out they drop after two sessions. Sometimes, the best thing you can do is to help them find a therapist who will move them toward resolving their underlying conflicts about their own self-worth, or a health and wellness coach who can help them improve their self-efficacy and develop a plan to reach their personal wellness vision one step at a time.

It will help you and your patients succeed in supporting their self-worth if you make it a point to "Reframe the task [at hand] from weight loss to self-care. People with a healthy sense of self-worth consistently and conscientious take care of their own health. Positive changes in thinking and behavior are fundamental to all psychotherapy treatments, but a sense of self-worth, which is a perceived and felt sense of self, cannot be meaningfully altered with CBT [Cognitive-Behavior Therapy] alone. When people perceive themselves as attractive or unattractive, intelligent or unintelligent, or adequate or inadequate, they live accordingly. Perception of self is experienced as reality and a negative self-perception robs many overweight patients of the faith in self to do what it takes to be healthy."[2]

Therapists and wellness coaches appreciate that lasting behavioral change is built upon a solid foundation of nonjudgmental awareness, consistent self-compassion and self-acceptance, and a well-defined wellness vision rooted in a person's individual values, plus a deliberate commitment to consistent, ongoing self-care. For patients, taking ownership of their own self-worth and taking the time to consider exactly what they want for themselves from a wellness standpoint can be empowering. This "internal locus of control" for wellness-related behaviors is what helps patients stay motivated and consistent with their healthful eating or activity regimen when outside forces interfere.

The fact is that "ego damage is harm to one's sense of self-worth, and many overweight patients come from ego-damaging families in which they developed a sense of inadequacy. Many learned to put the needs of others ahead of their own, leaving little time to attend to their own health. Their subsequent weight gain is then perceived as confirmation of their inadequacy."[3] Without appreciating that they might use food and overeating to try to care for themselves when they do not otherwise feel deserving of their own attention, patients may not recognize their troublesome eating behavior as part of their efforts to address an unmet need or manage feelings of inadequacy. They may feel trapped in a vicious, exhausting cycle. Because of this, experts recommend that in addressing eating and weight concerns, "We need treatments that include strategies to repair ego damage, enhance the sense of self-worth, and develop self-efficacy so that overweight patients can become the agents of change in their pursuit of well-being."[4] Such strategies are best found within an interdisciplinary model of patient care, which we discuss in later chapters.

In your professional interactions, you can model self-compassion by telling patients, "It seems like you've got a lot going on in your life, especially taking care of other people. I hope you're taking time for yourself." Or smile and say, "You know you are allowed to take care of yourself. You deserve it." The goal is to help patients believe that they are deserving of self-care and a healthy life regardless of their size. Once they believe that wholeheartedly, empowering self-talk and positive behavioral changes will likely follow more automatically.

---

Brain food for providers: What is the benefit of viewing patients' eating and weight struggles as self-care problems? Do you understand that the key to making permanent lifestyle changes is helping to increase feelings of self-worth and self-efficacy in a patient?

---

Brain food for patients: Do you have problems taking effective, ongoing care of your health? What did you learn about taking care of yourself growing up? Are you willing to focus on improving your total self-care as an actual goal rather than simply trying to lose weight?

---

### Beliefs

If what you've been doing with patients who have eating and weight concerns—focusing only on changing behavior—hasn't worked, it's time to try something different. Although we have machine-like parts of our bodies such as lungs, heart, and joints, we also have brains which are far less mechanistic. Beyond neurotransmitters and hormones, neural pathways and synapses, at the core of being sentient animals, we have a set of conscious or unconscious beliefs upon which our feelings and behaviors are predicated (whether we realize it or not).

In particular, we have cognitions regarding the value of certain foods, the activity of eating, weight ideals, and the importance of appearance. Beyond that, we have beliefs about what we deserve in life and our ability to achieve it. Isolating patients' behaviors from their beliefs and feelings about the above may be tempting, but it won't help you help them. Psychiatrist Aaron T. Beck, who pioneered Cognitive Therapy, now better known as Cognitive Behavior Therapy or CBT, was on to something when he began doing testing on how to conceptualize depression and had the realization that depressed patients' negative thoughts were the foundation of their depressive behaviors.[5] Dysregulated eaters, who are often chronic dieters, hold a slew of (conscious and unconscious) irrational, unhealthy beliefs about how their bodies got to where they are today and whether they can make them different tomorrow. Here are just a sampling of the beliefs they may possess which underlie their behaviors:

Beliefs about food: Foods are either good or bad, Food is the enemy, Food is love and comfort, I need to be in tight control of myself at all times around food, I am bad if I waste food, I should eat only nutritious foods, Food is the perfect reward, I can't trust myself around food, Eating "good" food makes me a good person and eating "bad" food makes me a bad person, If I had a better relationship with food, my life would be perfect, There is something defective about me that I can't have a sane relationship with food no matter how hard I try, Food is my best friend.

Beliefs about eating: I must finish all the food that's put in front of me, I better eat a lot now because tomorrow I may put myself on a diet, Eating is better than feeling emotional pain or discomfort, Eating is so psychologically painful that I wish I didn't need to do it, Hunger is scary, Eating fills the emptiness inside me, Eating is a great stress reliever, Feeling good or bad about myself is dependent on the foods I eat or avoid eating, I am being deprived if I can't eat whatever, whenever, or as much as I want, I'll never be any good at feeding myself, Other people eat what they want, so why can't I? I'm entitled to eat when I have had a hard day, Eating fills time and solves the problem of boredom, Eating is self-care, If I make or buy food, I must eat it all, I must only eat high-nutrient-density food, I must always eat from hunger and never for pleasure, Eating someone's food is a way to show I love them, Eating is better than feeling hurt.

Beliefs about weight, body size, or appearance: I must be thin or thinner to be lovable, I am fat and disgusting looking, People hate fat folks, Thin equals success and happiness, I should weigh myself every day if I want to be a comfortable weight, Weighing myself is the scariest part of my day, I'm a failure if I can't lose weight and keep it off, I don't trust my body to know what or how much it wants to eat, My fat body is something to be ashamed of, I love myself when I'm thin but not when I'm fat, My body will never look like I want it to, I hate my body no matter what size it is, Fat is ugly and thin is beautiful, It doesn't matter what positive attributes I have if I'm fat because no one will pay attention to them.

Imagine a prediabetic thirty-five-year-old female patient we'll call Liddy who is 5'1" and weighs 186 pounds, with a long history of dieting and regaining weight sitting across from you in your office. Let's say Liddy believes that food is the perfect reward and comfort after a stressful day, she's being unfairly deprived if she says no to the high-fat/high-calorie foods she enjoys, and she shouldn't need to lose weight for people to love her unconditionally. Now, we're not implying that these are rational beliefs, just that they are Liddy's and that she—like many people with unconscious beliefs—has no idea that they are holding her back from attaining health and happiness.

According to these beliefs, if you, her doctor or health care provider, tell her that she needs to lose weight, she's going to interpret that as you telling her she's not good enough or lovable enough as she is. Should you tell her to cut back on highly processed foods, she's going to feel deprived and unable to cope with her stressful day. What we have is you talking about her becoming healthier and her hearing only that she's not okay as she is and that life is about to become even more grim if she gives up her comfort and stress-relieving yummy food treats.

Now let's imagine another patient. At sixty-seven years, Al is 5'8", weighs close to 350 pounds (much of which he carries in his belly), and has had one knee replacement and suffered one heart attack. Al believes that it's a sin to waste food and not get your hard-earned money's worth, especially when he and his wife go out to dinner; eating is better than feeling emotional pain or discomfort; and no one has the right to tell him what he can eat and how much he should weigh because that's his business. While you're trying to help Al avoid another knee replacement and a second heart attack, he's thinking that you're crazy to advise him to waste uneaten food that he's paid good money for, you want him to be in emotional pain, and you're trying to control him by butting into his personal business.

This confusing dynamic, this common kind of miscommunication, this case of you not understanding where your patients are coming from and them being clueless that you're out to help, not harm, them, is frustrating and disheartening on both sides of the exam table. We're giving you extremes of beliefs about food, eating, and weight here, and we grant that not every patient presents with these kinds of irrational belief systems. Many more likely believe that they can take weight off but not keep it off; restricting food is a struggle that they don't want to do for the rest of their lives in any way, shape, or form; it's not fair that they have to stop eating foods they love when other people can eat them and not get fat; taking away food is taking away life's fun and pleasure; and the deprivation they're going to feel by giving up foods they love will make them so miserable, they'll be driven to, well, eat. These beliefs are not unusual, even among successful, high-achieving people, and patients do not need to present with a high BMI or weight in order to have them. Sadly, these beliefs are as common as a winter cold.

When you make suggestions or give advice to patients about what they can do to become healthier, ask permission first, and then make sure to check out their facial and body reactions. Do they fold their arms in front of their chest and nod pleasantly? Do they tense up or look away? It's fine to ask, "May I make an observation?" Or "I'm happy to make suggestions, but you know what's best for yourself, so don't feel you need to do something just because I think it might be a good idea," encouraging them to think for themselves and act wisely on their own behalf.

The above are only the beliefs that patients have about food, eating, and weight. In addition, they have what are called core beliefs, which form the foundation of their lives and dictate everything they say and do. Here are some core beliefs your patients may feel that may complicate the picture: I need to be perfect at eating or exercising or not even bother trying; I'm not a worthwhile person and don't deserve pleasure, health, or happiness; Life is a struggle, and eating well and exercising will be a struggle too; No one can tell me how to eat or what to do; People are always trying to manipulate or control me; I can't depend on anyone, so why bother to get support for eating better; I can't take care of my body, so why try; Everyone in my family dies young, so I probably will too; I'm a failure and a loser because my family always told me so, I never finish doing anything, so why bother starting; I'm not sure I'm worth taking care of; I need to live small, not take risks, not rock the boat.

We don't mean to make you feel helpless or despairing. On the contrary, we only want you to recognize that patients are brimming with unhealthy beliefs that can lead to what looks like self-sabotage or lack of concern for their health. When it comes to promoting lasting health behavior improvement, *these* are what you are up against as much as any medical conditions with which patients enter your office.

To learn more about rational and irrational eating, food, weight, and core beliefs, we refer you to *The Rules of "Normal" Eating* by Karen R. Koenig.

Brain food for providers: Are you aware or surprised that your patients have some or, more likely, many of the above beliefs? Does recognizing this help you understand why they struggle to make progress or attain consistency with resolving their eating and weight concerns?

Brain food for patients: Are you aware of having the beliefs listed above? Can you see how having them makes it difficult for you to change your eating habits? What steps will you take to make your beliefs more rational and healthy?

## HOW IS IT THAT PATIENTS CAN APPEAR SO GUNG HO AND EVEN DESPERATE TO IMPROVE THEIR EATING AND HEALTH, THEN TURN AROUND AND DO NEXT TO NOTHING TO HELP THEMSELVES?

### Mixed feelings

It often does seem truly mind-blowing how patients seem to have split personalities—hungering for better health, yet not doing a darned thing to achieve it. However, this pattern isn't indicative of mental illness, but of mental conflict: when patients say they want one thing and then go off and do the opposite, this is symptomatic of plain old, garden variety ambivalence. Other names for it are mixed, conflicting, opposing, or contradictory feelings. We want something and also want its opposite or, said in more psychological terms, we may desire and also fear something. And, sad to say, without psychology intervening, humans are hard-wired for fear to trump desire every time.

To understand the power of mixed feelings, let's look at examples of internal or intrapsychic conflicts outside the eating and weight arena. You want to plan a trip to visit your elderly parents because that is what a "good" son or daughter does, but your relationship with them is so strained that you always leave them vowing never to return. Or, you've been in practice for over forty years and feel burned out and tired of the same old grind, but also worry that if you retire, you won't know what to do with all your free time or be satisfied living with a steeply reduced income. Or, you wonder if you're overdoing it when you down a couple of glasses of wine at home after work, but don't wish to give them up because nothing else seems to decrease your stress so magically.

Get it? You want this and also you want that. Psychologically speaking, when our intent does not align with our actions, something is going on and we call that dynamic internal conflict. Most of us have mixed feelings about a great many things. This dynamic is pulling the strings when we waffle, procrastinate, or do something that benefits us for a while, then stop doing it. Sometimes we're aware of having these tugs within and sometimes we're not. Almost always, avoiding doing something we insist we want to do is a tell-tale sign that we have an internal conflict brewing. Our lives are filled with minor and major sets of ambivalent thoughts, and the best we can do is try to resolve as many as we can.

Now back to the subject of food and weight. Think about why patients might be ambivalent about giving up eating certain foods or having a particular identity (say, fat) that they've had their entire life. Consider how patients of high weight might want to do both: get fit, but dread going to the gym in form-fitting, flashy workout clothes; give up the pint of ice cream they share with their spouse while watching their favorite TV shows at night, yet feel upset about losing this intimate, cherished ritual; quit making a stop at McDonald's after work every day, but not know how else to de-stress and reward themselves before going home to take care of an invalid parent. Remember that, irrational creatures that we all are, many (if not most) of our decisions are made by our emotions and often without conscious deliberation.

There are a number of intrapsychic, generally unconscious conflicts that patients with eating problems often have that may derail them from attaining or sustaining their eating and weight goals.[6] "In fact, the internal struggle between the patient's desire to be healthy and her lack of faith in herself to do what it takes is reflected in the well-documented pattern of short-term weight loss followed by relapse that is independent of treatment models."[7] Although weight gain is often due to the body's metabolic reaction to restriction from dieting, sometimes it also reflects the ambivalence patients feel about giving up comfort foods or living in a smaller body.

- Conflicts about trying and failing (again and again)

Let's face it, you are probably not the first health care provider who has suggested or alluded to your patient eating more healthfully. Chances are good that many patients have been working on or avoiding working on (but still obsessing about) their relationship with food and weight for a long time, maybe even since childhood. That they don't eat healthfully or that they weigh more than they might prefer is not news to them. It is pretty much a post-it on their brains every minute of every day. Moreover, it's more than likely that they have dieted and even lost a substantial amount of weight one or more times.

Gallup polling reveals that "trying to lose weight is something most Americans can identify with. Two-thirds say they have made a serious effort to lose weight at least once in their life, including 25% saying they tried once or twice, 30% trying between three and 10 times, and 8% trying more than 10 times. Nearly three-quarters of women (73%) have ever attempted weight loss, with an average of seven attempts. By contrast, just over half of men (55%) have ever tried to lose weight, with the average trying fewer than four times."[8]

Unfortunately, the patient you see before you doesn't view herself as a success in shedding pounds (no matter how many she's shed and how often she's shed them), but as a failure for not keeping them shed. She is terrified of getting her hopes up about keeping her weight down and often fears disappointing others (again), depriving herself of foods she loves (again), obsessing about what she can and can't eat (again), dropping several dress sizes (again), and losing any number of pounds only to see the entire process reverse itself (again).

So, really, can you blame her for being a mite ambivalent upon embarking on the whole endeavor yet one more time? While you're focused on how she's going to become healthier, she's fixated on ending up exactly where she is now, with one more failure under her belt, and wondering why she should bother wasting her time and considerable effort. At best, she's ambivalent; at worst, she feels despairing and helpless.

- Conflicts about giving up food for comfort and pleasure

Imagine if suddenly all your comforts were taken away—no more TV or iPhone, Pinterest, hobbies, Barcalounger, get-away cabin in the mountains, friends, or pet Pug. You would undoubtedly feel utterly lost and bereft. Even if having every one of these things had an obvious downside (though we can't think of any for a Barcalounger), you would still feel their loss because of the sheer enjoyment they bring you.

Now imagine if one of the major pleasures—no, make that the only pleasure—in your life was food, glorious food. Or if you believed that eating was the glue that kept your life together because food made sure you were never bored or lonely, sad or anxious. Remove the glue and you imagine your whole life falling apart. That is what it is like for many dysregulated eaters when they imagine giving up the foods they love (or even eating them in smaller quantities than they're used to). Sure they want to be healthier and slimmer, but it's difficult for them to reconcile these lofty goals at the expense of suffering such perceived catastrophic loss.

Hyperbole, you might think. Not really. This is what your patients are feeling. This is what the authors of this book felt when we thought of giving up food for comfort and pleasure. Emotional eaters fervently wish to believe that they can eat normally—after all other people seem to have acquired the knack—but are terrified nonetheless. And this is what produces their conflicting feelings: wanting more than anything in their lives to give up using food for comfort and pleasure and just as strongly living in terror of giving it up.

- Conflicts about deserving health, happiness, and feeling positive about themselves

We are all encouraged when people tell us that they wish to be healthy and enjoy a happy life. We are fooled because many of the people who say this are fooling themselves due to not recognizing the truth. They think they want all these things (who wouldn't?), but deep down don't feel deserving of them. Not all of us had joyful childhoods where our parents loved us unconditionally and wanted the best for us so that we internalized their love and caring and now love and care well for ourselves.

True, some people who were abused or neglected get out there and try to prove their parents wrong by succeeding, most often through overachieving. Some of them may even end up ratcheting up their self-esteem so that they no longer need to prove anything to anyone. But others were put down so many times that they carry deep within them the conviction that there is something terribly, irrevocably wrong with them, that they are defective, and that they don't deserve either a good life or the best in life.

If patients are conflicted about self-worth, how can they achieve success and, often the more difficult task of maintaining it? Sometimes they do succeed: they eat better and exercise regularly and their triglyceride levels and LDL plummet, they lower their hemoglobin A1C and start to get their diabetes under control, and maybe even enjoy the thrill of running a 5K race with friends or family. These accomplishments spring from the part of themselves that wishes to believe that they're worthy, so they allow themselves the gift of success.

But then doubt creeps in, triggered by the discomfort of unfamiliarity about feeling deserving. "I'm fooling everyone, including myself. Soon people will see right through me and know that I'm a fraud and that I don't deserve all these good feelings and kind words." And so begins the abrupt or gradual descent into perceived undeservedness and the thoughts of "Gee, I guess Mom was right and I won't amount to anything. I'm too lazy to even cook a decent dinner for myself" or "Dad always said I can't stick to anything and who am I to prove him wrong. Look at me, I haven't been for a run in weeks. My career may be in great shape, but my eating habits are a mess."

Many high achievers, raised in families in which there was tremendous overt as well as subtle pressure to succeed, do so, but they still feel as if they don't deserve it. The name of this phenomenon is "The Imposter Syndrome," a term first coined by Suzanne Imes, Ph.D., and Pauline Rose Clance, Ph.D., in the 1970s. Also called intellectual self-doubt, this phenomenon, which makes it difficult or even impossible to accept success or achievement, including weight loss and "normal" eating, is "generally accompanied by anxiety, and, often depression. It is one of the causes of the internal dissonance that some people who've lost weight feel and one of the reasons the weight comes back on."[9]

Thus the yo-yo dynamic, the revolving door, the arduous climb to the top of the mountain and the awful, shocking, rapid slide back down. Most of your patients may have no idea they feel undeserving or even uncomfortable with their success, but their patterns belie their pretense of worthiness and happiness, whether they know it or not.

- Conflicts about emotional and sexual intimacy

Intimacy is generally portrayed and thought of as a heavenly, blissful state: we trust, open our hearts, expose our authenticity, surrender to vulnerability, lean on others, and ecstatically merge with another human being. But that's only the upside of closeness. The downside is the fear that most of us have experienced: of lost intimacy through physical or emotional abandonment (intentional or accidental), betrayal, or rejection; of our vulnerability being manipulated or used against us; of our emotional supports being stripped away and of falling flat on our faces; or of isolation and perpetual loneliness. It should surprise no one that we are frightened of intimacy because it holds within it the seeds of its loss.

What does intimacy have to do with eating and weight? Plenty. Odd as it may sound, some patients may use their size as a barrier to intimacy. It can (if they let it) reduce the number of people who: will ask them out, wish to have intimate physical relations with them, and take the time to unwrap the cocoon in which they've swathed themselves. This isn't because they are not wonderful people worthy of love or intimacy. It's just the way our fat-phobic, thin-obsessed society operates and the way that people with body image issues, particularly those at the higher end of the weight spectrum, often perceive themselves.

Love and intimacy are always a double-edged sword. Being large can function like the keep out sign on a teenager's door, especially in the arena of sexuality. Let's face it, sex means physical closeness and maybe even emotional closeness. It's both a metaphoric and real undressing and laying bare of oneself.

Moreover, many people of higher weight report feeling more comfortable with their sexuality when they're thinner. Some fear that they will act on those feelings. With intensified sexual feelings and being hit on more often due to conforming to cultural attractiveness standards comes the possibility of cheating in a monogamous relationship or being super-sexually active (what is judgmentally called promiscuous) as a single person. This is frightening to some people, men and women alike. So, sometimes to not act on their erotic impulses or not act on them as they did the last time they slimmed down, they end up putting the weight back on, which allows them to rationalize a return to a more comfortable asexual status quo.

- Conflicts about being controlled by others

You easily may be able to distinguish someone caring about you from someone trying to control you, but, we assure you, to many people, they feel like one and the same. It all depends on your upbringing. If your parents were my-way-or-the-highway kind of folks and schooling was rigid and built on top-down dictums, you may be sick and tired of being told what to do. When parents are domineering and demanding and children have little or no say in most matters, they can build up a serious head of steam about being told what to do—or worse, being lectured, badgered, bossed around, and punished for doing what they want. What may emerge is someone who will fight against being told what to do and will go out of his or her way to ignore or do the opposite of what is expected—even when it's clearly not in their best interest.

We know it sounds irrational that patients would rebel against what's best for them, but this is what happens—too often, unfortunately. There you are expressing your wish that a patient become a little more active because you actually like him and want him to live long and prosper. And he's hearing you as yet one more person who believes he can't think for or take care of himself, one more lecturer about what he *should* do and *needs* to do, one more authority figure out to control his life. A related conflict is that people may fear that successful behavior change in the present will increase their vulnerability to criticism if success in childhood was met with criticism from others (perhaps by a competitive parent or sibling). In this way, success becomes both a hoped-for and dreaded occurrence.

Clinically, what's happening here is that the patient is taking an old, interpersonal problem and re-enacting it in the present, making you the hated authority figure, a dynamic psychology calls transference. Another dynamic that occurs is that patients internalize an old interpersonal conflict and it becomes a current intrapsychic one: when their inner voice is urging them to broil a nice piece of fish rather than eat packaged fried filets for dinner or not to finish the bag of cookies they're devouring while watching TV, they feel bullied and refuse do it.

These are strange dynamics, to be sure, re-enacting old interpersonal battles around food, exercise, and self-care when the battlefield is one's psyche. They sound like this: "Go to the gym and you'll feel better," challenged by "I know I should but I don't feel like it." Or "You know that if you bring that bag of malted milk balls home, you're going to eat them all," challenged by "So what, I'll eat them if I want to." Or "You'll feel better tomorrow if you go to bed rather than stay up and eat ice cream," challenged by "I'm sick of being told what to do. I'm entitled to eat whatever I want."

When you sense that a patient wants to do something—start biking more, buy a treadmill, cut down on eating out at restaurants, or buy more nutritious foods—but that he or she is having difficulty taking action, you can always say something like "It's not unusual to have forces that make you want to move forward in taking care of yourself and forces that want to hold you back. Like many people, you may have mixed feelings about all you feel you need to do to get healthier."

To learn about more conflicts that your patients might have around food and weight, read Karen R. Koenig's *Starting Monday—Seven Keys to a Permanent,*

*Positive Relationship with Food.* It's all about these conflicts and how to resolve them.

---

Brain food for providers: After reading about internal conflicts, do you have a deeper comprehension of why your patients seem to sabotage their own best efforts, taking one step forward, two steps back? How does recogniz-ing these conflicts give you more compassion for your patients? How might you help them recognize and resolve these mixed feelings?

---

Brain food for patients: Do you have any of the above conflicts? Which ones are the greatest barriers to resolving your food and weight concerns? Do you feel more compassion for yourself now that you understand that what looks like self-sabotage in the health and wellness arena is often a symptom of an internal conflict? Who could you speak with about them to get full resolution?

---

## WHAT MAKES IT SO HARD FOR SOME CLIENTS TO MANAGE THEIR LIVES MORE THOUGHTFULLY AND HEALTHFULLY?

### Life skills

In order to succeed at anything, we can't depend on sheer luck, hope, or prayers. We need skills. The abilities we require to live fully functional lives as adults are called life skills and are defined by the World Health Organization as "abilities for adaptive and positive behavior that enable individuals to deal effectively with the demands and challenges of everyday life."[10] Life skills fall under categories like taking care of your health, managing stress and emo-tions, living purposefully and in balance, handling relationships, and problem solving and critical thinking.[11]

Life skills are not unlike occupational skills in that they provide us with tools to get a job done well. Sadly, however, we have no such curriculum, practice arena or exam for life skills. We simply toss people into the sea of life and they either sink or swim. Moreover, we can't assume that because people have excel-lent occupational or social skills, that they also possess top-notch life skills. When patients with eating and weight concerns come to see you, you might make assumptions about their life skills based on their occupational skills—she's a high-powered attorney, he's a prosperous real estate mogul, she successfully raised four great kids single-handedly, or he received an award for Principal of the Year. Think of the exceptional people you know in your field who are respected and honored, but who live in a state of perpetual struggle and dissatisfaction because they lack life skills or what you might even call "common sense."

Effective life skills don't suddenly and magically develop on their own, but need to be taught and practiced. If our role models modeled and taught us effective life skills, how fortunate we were. If what we saw and learned was mediocre, well, maybe we make do and, if we're lucky, pick up what we missed along the way. But what if our role models had very little functionality and what we came away with in the life skills department was bupkis? What then? How do we cope with life? There are a number of life skill areas in which patients often have deficits which impact their ability to eat well and exercise consistently. Recognizing what they're missing will help you be more compassionate toward them and help you guide them toward support services.

- Physical self-care

This skill can be compromised if, as discussed earlier, we are not competently cared for by our parents or if they didn't model proper self-care for us. You can't expect a patient who never was served fresh vegetables to start craving them because health guidelines now say that they're good for him or her. Or one who was given take-out or frozen dinners every night in childhood to suddenly know how to or enjoy cooking. Moreover, eating well is not just about what patients feed themselves but also about why they eat. If they had parents who used food for comfort ("I know I shouldn't have a second piece of cake, but I'm so lonely since your father left us") and diversion ("There's nothing on TV, so, hey, kids, let's go for ice cream"), they will need to recognize and change these habitual patterns in order to take better care of their health.

Physical self-care isn't only about food and exercise, however. It's about patients viewing their bodies as precious objects and taking commensurate care of them. Patients first need to learn *why* they would wish to value their bodies and only then *how* to do it through healthy and "normal" eating and physical activity. Remember that this is unchartered territory for many patients, so be careful not to make the assumption that they want or know how to care for their bodies. Many don't have a clue.

- Managing stress and emotions

Consider that "emotional eating is considered a risk factor for eating disorders and an important contributor to obesity and its associated health problems. Linear regression analyses found that proneness to boredom and difficulties in emotion regulation simultaneously predicted inappropriate eating behavior, including eating in response to boredom, other negative emotions, and external cues."[12] Managing emotions is perhaps the major life skill that dysregulated eaters lack. They don't know how to prevent stress from building up, make choices which avoid or lessen it, or what to do when they experience too much of it. Moreover, some patients, through temperament or upbringing (or both), see most of life as stressful. Whereas some folks might view changing jobs as challenging or exciting, other patients view it as worrisome and terrifying. Whereas some might think that living alone is freeing because they're beholden to no one, others may find it scary and overwhelming to take care of all the major and minor details of life themselves.

Moreover, many patients, particularly those who are depressed, find it mega-angst provoking to go grocery shopping or cook meals for themselves or others. For various reasons, they are uncomfortable with what they perceive as too much responsibility for themselves; rather, they're desperate for people to take care of them. Explaining to someone which aisles to avoid in the supermarket or how to read a label is pointless if all the time he or she is thinking, "I hate grocery shopping almost as much as I hate cooking. It's too stressful. I can't do it. It's too much work."

Some patients lead lives that are brimming with stress from childrearing, taking caring of elderly parents, and demanding jobs. Unfortunately, brainstorming with them about how to reduce stress in their lives actually may cause them more agita because they fear they'll fail at what you suggest. Eating is cheap, quick, and easy as a relaxant compared to finding or paying a baby sitter in order to go to the gym or take a meditation class. Eating feels less taxing than taking a walk during a lunch break or when energy is flagging mid-afternoon. People who are easily stressed or who have (intentionally or unconsciously) set up their lives to be stress filled want instant relief and are not thinking about what they're doing to their bodies with food other than chilling them out momentarily.

Managing emotions is another sad affair. Brené Brown, social work professor at the University of Houston, popular TED talk presenter, and best-selling author of *Daring Greatly* and *The Gifts of Imperfection*, "asked hundreds of people to list all the emotions that you understand in yourself. The average number was three: happy, sad and pissed off. We don't have a full emotional lexicon."[13] Unfortunately, many of us are more familiar with emoticons than with actual real-life emotions. If patients can't identify *what* they feel, how in the world will they know what will make them feel better (other than food, of course)?

When we do think of feelings, too often we feel fear and confusion. We think that emotions are pesky annoyances, trying to drag us down or bum us out. We have no use or time for them: the heck with *feelings*, we need to get on with the action of life. This is the attitude that Western culture has taught us about our emotional lives, so it's not surprising that many patients are out of touch with feelings and have no earthly idea of what to do with discomfiting ones. It seems to them like a no-brainer: experience internal distress (never mind identifying exactly what the emotion is) or grab some cookies. Duh! Importantly, some people feel that if they are experiencing negative emotions or difficult feelings, or if a situation is difficult or suboptimal, that they must be doing something wrong. How freeing (or terrifying) it is when they learn and accept that imperfection is an expected, normal part of a life well-lived!

Unless patients become more skilled at preventing and managing stress and identifying, experiencing, and handling intense or difficult feelings effectively, no amount of nutrition counseling is going to stop them from emotional eating. After all, food-seeking is a biological imperative. Emotional management, not so much. Knowing what you're feeling and what to do with whatever emotions come up can make all the difference between mindless emotional eating as an ineffective attempt to self-soothe and healthy stress management behaviors. "As predicted [in a NIH study], emotional awareness moderated the link between urgency and binge eating."[14] In his book, *Emotional Intelligence*, Daniel Goleman, Ph.D., explains that "emotions that simmer beneath the threshold of awareness can have a powerful impact on how we perceive and react, even though we have no idea they are at work."[15] Goleman cites research by Leon et al., indicating that "emotional deficits—particularly a failure to tell distressing feelings from one another and to control them—were found to be key among the factors leading to eating disorders."[16]

Feel free to tell patients that they might want to consider an alternate approach if they've been trying to eat better by using willpower alone. Then explain that they, instead, might need to enhance their life skills because none of us were born or brought up to have all the skills we need to manage life well. Make it okay to have challenging life skill areas. Tell patients, "You know, we learn so many skills in school, or when we're new to a sport, but sometimes the hardest skills to learn are the ones we were never taught: how to balance work and play or take care of our emotions."

- Self-regulation

We are not automatic regulating machines like our thermostats which flip on or off and up or down a smidge as needed. We need to regulate ourselves, and not just with eating, but this is often easier said than done. Unfortunately, most, if not all, dysregulated eaters have similar "What's enough?" problems in other areas of their lives: work, play, parenting, sleep, spending, stress, etc. In order to self-regulate effectively, patients need to be in touch with what they are feeling, not only with food but also by sensing sufficiency and adequacy.

If they grew up in families in which their feelings were ignored or invalidated (which many dysregulated eaters did), they may well be unable to register and recognize body signals for when to start or stop eating. Instead, they go from one extreme (dieting) to the other (bingeing or overeating), ignore both hunger and satiation signals, and swing from spending hours at the gym to whiling away hours in front of the TV or computer.

Self-regulation, which is rooted in sensing emotional and physical signals, is key to "normal" eating (which will be discussed later in this chapter). In fact, without this skill, "normal" eating cannot and will not occur. "Behavioral theory suggests that treatments that increase participants' use of self-regulatory skills and/or their feelings of ability (self-efficacy) will improve exercise and nutrition behaviors. Despite limited evidence, higher autonomous motivation, self-efficacy, and self-regulation skills emerged as the best predictors of beneficial weight and physical activity outcomes." Moreover, "There was evidence of carry-over, or generalization, of both self-regulation and self-efficacy changes from an exercise context to an eating context."[17]

- Critical thinking, goal setting, and problem solving

Ask many folks what critical thinking is, and they may well be uncertain and say, "Always telling people what's wrong with them." Critical thinking is not exactly a household term, but it should be. If we are not taught how to think clearly and rationally in childhood and don't learn how in school, where would we develop this must-have capacity to discern what works and what doesn't?

The fact is that many patients lead with their feelings, let their hearts overrule their heads, and don't consider follow through, consequences, or cause and effect. The most important decisions of their lives are made this way—who they marry, how they vote, and the way they raise their children. If they don't think rationally about these choices, how can you expect them to apply rationality to eating or exercise? Who among us hasn't heard folks say, "Oh, I don't go to the doctor (or the hospital or the dentist). I hate going there." As if whether we like or dislike something is the sole arbiter for doing it or not.

As to goal setting, many patients either weren't taught how to set and reach goals, had no one to model this process for them, or had such pressure to achieve, improve, and win at all costs that they might be afraid to move forward; or they're tired of striving all the time and now simply want to sit back and watch life go by. They even may feel that their major goal is to have no goals. Either way, health care professionals would do well not to assume that their patients know how to set doable, realistic, concrete, chunked down goals and stay motivated enough to reach them incrementally.

One caveat on goals is that many patients who've struggled with food and the scale are super wary about setting eating and exercise goals because they see the process as a sure-fire way to fail. If patients don't want to set eating or weight goals, please do not push behavioral goals until they are more ready for change. This means they will need to acknowledge, identify, and resolve whatever internal, likely unconscious, mixed feelings they have about success (see above conflicts). Mainly, they just don't want to fail again, and are better off identifying and evaluating their beliefs, thoughts, and feelings about their circumstances rather than establishing quantitative objectives or target dates. Moreover, they may say yes to goals because they think that's what you want to hear, rather than goals springing from what they wish to do. They want to feel that success is possible, but after multiple failures, they can't help but look to their experience which laughs in the face of their hopes and dreams.

Regarding problem solving, many patients will agree that they'd like to develop better eating and activity habits—but believe they must do it by themselves. They strongly and wrongly believe that doing something on their own is better than succeeding with help. It may sound silly (no man is an island and all), but this is what a great many dysregulated eaters (and others) think.

The idea of meeting with a dietician or working with an exercise trainer gets translated in their minds into meaning, "I guess I'm a failure because I can't solve my eating and weight problems on my own." They're so ashamed that they can't manage their food concerns that they think asking for help will make things worse and only view success as something they've achieved single-handedly. They honestly believe that if they get help, they're not really earning success.

They may be slightly more open to help when it's normalized and universalized by you, the practitioner—for example, if you were to say that you hardly expect patients to resolve these problems on their own and that there's nothing in the least unusual about seeking or benefiting from support. You might even suggest that if you were in their shoes, soliciting help is exactly what you'd do. It's fine to say, "I think we all need help on some things. I know I do."

One more factor, which is perhaps more attitude than skill, is having a "growth" versus a "fixed" mindset. Stanford University developmental psychologist Carol Dweck, Ph.D., writes about them in her book *Mindset: The New Psychology of Success*.[18] People with a fixed mindset see themselves and their attributes or inadequacies as more or less permanent—they're good at some things and bad at others, outgoing or shy, lovable or unlovable. They view their successes as a "reflection of their more or less immutable gifts or talents" and their failures as a "reflection of unchangeable deficits and weaknesses." So many dysregulated eaters have this kind of fixed mindset: they're either one way or another and mostly do not feel good enough about themselves. Desperate to succeed, they're thrilled and relieved when they do and feel awful when they don't, as if failure confirms what they knew all along—there's something permanently defective about them.

Fixed-mindset thinkers might say to themselves, "I don't exercise because I'm lazy." A growth-mindset thinker would say, "I need to develop better strategies for getting myself to exercise because the ones I've been using aren't working very well." "People with a growth mindset explain their successes entirely differently, as the result of conscious, actively chosen behaviors and strategies." They attribute their success to having practiced a lot, made healthy choices, or thought more rationally. "When growth-mindset thinkers fail, they don't blame their intrinsic inadequacies but look for different strategies to succeed as in 'I could try. . . .'"

Of course, it's not your job to teach life skills to patients. It is your job, however, to recognize how deficits in these skill sets strongly and inevitably will impair patients' ability to take better care of their health for the long term. Moreover, by understanding that we all have some form of life-skill deficits, you might have more compassion for your patients (and yourself) and less frustration when they feel overwhelmed with expectations or don't follow your advice consistently. The best you can do is to take these patients as they are and try to nudge them along with your caring and compassion—and encouragement about baby steps. To learn more about life skills and their impact on food and weight, we refer you to *Outsmarting Overeating—Boost Your Life Skills, End Your Food Problems* by Karen R. Koenig. You may also refer to the training modules on Dr. O'Mahoney's website at http://www.deliberatelifewellness.com.

## WHAT MAKES A "NORMAL" EATER?

Most people use the terms nutritious/healthy eaters and "normal" eaters interchangeably when they actually have quite different meanings. As you learned in Chapter 4, on one end of the spectrum, dysregulated eaters seek food when they're not hungry (mindlessly, emotionally, and compulsively) and often eat past full or satisfaction (overeating or binge eating). On the other, they deprive and deny themselves nourishment or food pleasure when they are eating restrictively (via diets). They fail to regulate their intake so that they eat just enough most of the time—to maintain a comfortable weight, derive sensory pleasure, feel satisfied with food or how wonderful it feels in their bodies, and nourish themselves effectively.

"Normal" eaters generally base their food intake on a combination of two specific areas of information: appetite cues related to hunger, cravings, food enjoyment, and fullness/satisfaction as well as rational thinking about food and weight. You may be wondering what's with the quotation marks around the word "normal." They indicate a set of internal guidelines (conscious or unconscious) on which food consumption is predicated—to (1) eat mostly when you're hungry, (2) choose foods that satisfy you and feel good in your body, (3) eat with awareness and with an eye toward pleasure, and (4) stop eating when you're full or satisfied. "Normal" could also be called regulated eating, but that sounds more like the timed feedings that pediatrician Dr. Benjamin Spock might have advised.

Nutritious eaters, on the other hand, choose foods exclusively for their nutritive value and are not necessarily "normal" eaters. Think of eaters as coming in four varieties: (1) "normal" and nutritious, (2) non-"normal" and nutritious, (3) "normal" and non-nutritious, and (4) non-"normal" and non-nutritious.[19]

| "normal" and nutritious | non-"normal" and nutritious |
|---|---|
| "normal" and non-nutritious | non-"normal" and non-nutritious |

Non-"normal," non-nutritious eaters listen neither to their appetite signals nor care about eating what we would call a healthful diet. Non-"normal," nutritious eaters disregard appetite cues, but choose mostly foods that will nourish their bodies effectively. They may nosh mindlessly on fruits and veggies all day long, never pass the refrigerator without taking "healthy" food from it, and ingest huge amounts of foods that are nutritious but that make their bodies uncomfortable. "Normal," non-nutritious eaters eat according to appetite but eschew nutrition guidelines. They may leave some of their fried calamari or hot fudge sundae and eat only half a white-bread sandwich with processed meat and gobs of mayo because they're full. And, finally, "normal," nutritious eaters consume food according to appetite and focus on choosing mostly foods of high nutritive value.

Obviously, you would like to move your patients in the direction of eating both "normally" and nutritiously. The best rule of thumb is to guide patients toward becoming "normal" eaters first and, when those behaviors have taken root—and only then—encourage them to tweak their food intake to gradually become more nutritious. If they move toward nutrition too quickly, it will feel like a diet (restrictive and deprivational) and they're all too likely to rebel with rebound eating, consuming large quantities of non-nutritive food and falling back into old habits, failing to attune to internal appetite signals.

As you already pretty much know what constitutes a nutritious eater, let us focus on the profile of a "normal" eater. Whether they eat three balanced meals a day—morning, noon and night—or six small meals throughout the day, they follow their appetite signals for hunger, craving, food enjoyment, fullness, and satisfaction most of the time. They may do this consciously or unconsciously, whether eating alone or with people, whether they're stressed or relaxing, and whether they're at home or on vacation. The crucial point is that the locus of control over their eating is within them, not based on some diet plan or program.

They plan ahead so as not to be starving for long periods of time and don't care for that bloated, full feeling. Tasty satisfaction from a holiday meal brings a smile to their faces, but so do many other activities, and their main source of pleasure in life is not food. Sometimes they put off eating because they're too busy, and other times they eat when they're not particularly hungry because food will not be accessible when they might be later on. They are not perfect eaters, as if there were such a thing, and don't even think about perfection. They are as likely to occasionally overeat as under-eat but pay these behaviors no mind.

They believe that food is mostly for nourishment and occasionally for pleasure, and may have concern for their weight, but don't base their eating on it. If their weight decreases, they don't think, "Oh, boy, I can eat more," and if it increases, they don't panic that they need to rush into diet mode. If they do weigh themselves, they don't give the number on the scale the power to make or break their day. They eat without shame, and may be interested in what their dining companions are eating, but without such interest causing self-consciousness about their own food choice. They don't think a cookie will solve their emotional problems, but occasionally seek tasty food just for the pleasure of it.

Understand that these "normal" eaters are not saints or paragons of virtue and may have multitudes of other problems. They may drink, do drugs, yell at their children, scam their employers, be rude to their neighbors, run afoul of the law, and be no one you'd ever want to talk with for more than a few minutes. The one problem they don't have is with food.

Chapters 7 and 8 will teach you how to work with dysregulated eaters and point them in the direction of "normal" eating by getting them the help they need.

Brain food for providers: In treating patients with eating and weight concerns, can you see how lacking effective life skills makes it very difficult or even impossible for them to make the changes they need in their lives to improve or sustain their eating and health? How does this increase your empathy toward them? How does it change your approach to helping them?

Brain food for patients: Which of the above life skills are you missing or do you perform barely adequately? Do you have a better understanding now of how lacking effective life skills has made it difficult for you to take better consistent care of yourself? What steps can you take to improve them?

Providers, try . . .

1. Changing your conversation with patients from a weight to a health focus.
2. Getting a sense of what patients believe about food, eating, weight, and their appearance.
3. Gently pointing out how having healthier (i.e., rational) beliefs will help them eat more healthfully and take more consistent care of their bodies.
4. Fostering the healthy or realistic beliefs of your patients (which may well mean understanding and changing your own belief system on eating, fitness, and weight).
5. Eschewing use of "good" and "bad" when talking about food and replacing these words with "more and less nutritious," taking the focus off morality and putting it where it belongs, on health.
6. Gently encouraging patients to speak kindly and compassionately about their bodies no matter what their size.
7. Helping patients focus on improving the life skills they lack.
8. Helping patients identify mixed feelings about consistently eating better, getting fit, and improving health care habits.
9. Identifying eating disorder therapists in your community who understand internal conflicts that your patients may have about food and the scale and referring your patients to them.

Patients, try . . .

1. Listing your beliefs about eating, food, weight, and appearance and determining which are rational and irrational. Use *The Rules of "Normal" Eating* to reframe beliefs from irrational to rational.
2. Feeling proud that you're trying to change beliefs rather than feeling ashamed of what you've believed.

3. Exploring and reframing your unhealthy beliefs, improving your life skills, and resolving your mixed feelings about food and your body with a psychotherapist or coach.

4. Digging deeply within yourself and identifying what your mixed feelings are about food, weight, eating, and appearance, and reading *Starting Monday* to resolve them.

5. Instead of feeling ashamed that you have mixed feelings, life skill deficits, or unhealthy beliefs, feeling proud that you're trying hard to improve in these areas.

6. Letting your doctor or health care provider know that you're aware of conflicting feelings around food and weight and that you're working to resolve them.

7. Using the self-assessment in *Outsmarting Overeating* by Karen R. Koenig to identify which life skills would help you have a better relationship with food and your body.

# Why Don't Patients Listen to Me about Eating Better?

## *(Why Don't I Listen to Myself?)*

- How doctors who have eating and weight concerns feel about treating patients with similar issues
- How explicit versus implicit provider attitudes about high-weight patients differ
- Research on weight prejudice and fat stigma in the medical professions
- The impact of health professionals' weight on their treatment of higher-weight patients
- Reactions of providers toward higher-weight patients
- How patients view providers of high weight
- Eight simple strategies to help patients with eating and weight concerns

If, as a provider, you and food aren't on the best of terms, you may be wondering how you can possibly approach or treat your patients' eating problems effectively. You may concur with the saying "Physician, heal thyself" and believe that unless you can manage your relationship with food, you have no right telling others how to do so. Sadly, you may even think that unless you're the poster doc for fit and trim, you have no business advising your patients about eating or exercise.

The good news is that if you believe the above to be true, you'd be wrong! Think about psychotherapists with emotional scars who may not have completely healed from their own traumas, yet do wondrous healing with their patients who are trauma victims and survivors. Or family therapists who may have had or still have terrible relationships with their dysfunctional families who are, nevertheless, considered tops in their field. Not for nothing are those in the psychological professions called wounded healers. They know that many patients don't expect them to be models of perfection in every aspect of life. In fact, sometimes patients are relieved that clinicians can relate to their problems and, therefore, are not looking down on and sitting in judgment of them. When this happens, patients take providers off their pedestals and place them where they belong—sitting squarely in the chair across from them.

The even better news is that, not only can you help patients resolve their eating and weight concerns without having fixed your own (by supporting patients in becoming more nonjudgmental, self-compassionate, and empowered on their journey to "normal" and nutritious eating), but these success-promoting habits will likely rub off on you. The key is not to widen the divide between you and your patients, or to pretend it doesn't exist, but for you to join with them in spirit on their quest to attain and maintain a sane and healthy relationship with food and their bodies.

## WHAT DO DOCTORS AND HEALTH CARE PROVIDERS FEEL WHEN THEY HAVE A POOR RELATIONSHIP WITH FOOD, LIVE WITH HIGH WEIGHTS, AND ARE NOT FIT AS A FIDDLE?

They feel pretty much the same as everyone else does—but more so. Some of you may be unhappy and frustrated that you do too much emotional, stress, and mindless eating, fail to exercise enough, and have trouble keeping away from high-calorie and high-fat foods. You may harbor deep shame about this failure along with self-contempt that, despite all your achievements, your eating goals continue to elude you. You may think about food and worry about your high weight more than you'd like to admit, keep promising loved ones you'll take better care of yourself, or try to put these concerns out of your mind and pretend you're perfectly healthy. Everyone or no one may know how badly you feel about your relationship with food and the scale.

If you're like most people who struggle with eating dysregulation or a higher-than-comfortable weight, you've probably dieted as much as your patients have and gone through spurts of weight loss followed by gradual weight gain. With all you know about the human body, you're still probably convinced that you failed at dieting, rather than that diets have failed you. You, too, have probably been brainwashed by our diet-obsessed culture and have not known what to do to resolve your own eating problems.

But, unlike most people of high weight, you're paid to spend (at least a portion of) your days telling people how to eat healthfully, exercise more, manage stress, and get fit. You may even wonder how all this treatment focus on food and exercise came about. One day you entered medical or nursing school to heal the sick and save lives, and the next, it seems, you're trying to persuade your patients to count carbs and climb stairs. We suspect that this isn't what you signed up for.

Looking around, you may see only those in your profession who seem to stay magically trim, or who find the time to run 10K races or hike and bike every weekend. They seem to be paragons of self-control and you look at yourself and simply don't know how they do it. The fact is that most medical professionals don't do very well with keeping their bodies fit, according to statistics.

- In the United States, "roughly 6 in 10 doctors and nurses today are overweight or obese, a level approaching that in the general population."[1]
- Simon Stevens, National Health Services England chief executive, has gone so far as to admonish doctors and nurses in England to slim down, citing "700,000 NHS staff classed as overweight or obese," and saying, "It is hard to talk about how important this [issue] is if we don't get our act together."[2]
- A University of Maryland School of Nursing study found that "55% of the 2,103 female nurses they surveyed were obese, citing job stress and the effect on sleep of long, irregular hours as the cause."[3]
- In a Harvard Nurses Health Study, "70% of the respondents were either overweight or obese—with 40% falling into the latter category."[4]
- Keith-Thomas Ayoob, associate professor at Albert Einstein College of Medicine, speaks wisely on the subject: "Nurses are just as susceptible to health problems as the rest of society. Before we were health professionals, we were real people. Just because we became health professionals doesn't mean we stopped being members of regular society with all the problems that go along with it. It illustrates that knowledge alone isn't always enough to produce behavioral changes."[5]

This last statement is a very telling one that is worth repeating: "Knowledge alone isn't always enough to produce behavioral changes." In addition to knowledge, doctors and health care providers could use more self-understanding and self-compassion—and it wouldn't hurt to learn more about how psychology can help resolve eating problems.

---

Brain food for providers: How do you feel about your weight? If you have a higher weight, what's your assessment of how diets have helped or hurt you in the long term? How do you feel speaking with patients about eating, weight, and fitness issues if you do not perceive yourself to be a role model for them? Do your food struggles make you feel more or less sympathetic to patients of high weights?

---

## WHY WOULD I HAVE ANY FEELINGS ABOUT MY PATIENTS, NO MATTER WHAT THEIR WEIGHT, OTHER THAN WANTING TO HEAL THEM?

Why? Because you're human. We have all sorts of beliefs and feelings about people, some of which are explicit and some of which are implicit. "Explicit attitudes and stereotyping operate in a conscious mode and are exemplified by traditional, self-report measure of these constructs. Implicit attitudes and stereotypes, in contrast, are evaluations and beliefs that are automatically activated by the mere presence (actual or symbolic) of the attitude object. They commonly function in an unconscious fashion."[6] Explicit beliefs are those we know we have, while implicit ones are the ones we don't know we have.

This lack of awareness is why we may say (and truly believe) that we feel one way, yet have our behavior betray us. For example, you might insist that you are comfortable with your body but still choose not to look in a full length mirror after a shower if you can help it. Or you might think you believe that women can be as good in math and science as men are but be disappointed that your son chose a female adviser while writing his Ph.D. dissertation in astrophysics.

Living in our fat-phobic, thin-obsessed culture that has been sending us the same message for decades—fat is bad, fat is unhealthy, fat is ugly, fat is dangerous, and fat is fatal—how could anyone possibly think we would escape being brainwashed? We may sound as if we're overstating our case here, but we as health care providers have been programmed as deeply as the general public into believing that fat is one of the worst things you can be on the planet.

If you're totally honest with yourself, how *do* you feel about people of size— a.k.a. fat people? What crosses your mind when you watch them walk down the street or take a seat on a bus? What thought pops into your head unbidden when you see them food shopping, eating in a restaurant, or sitting at your own dining room table? (Or, heaven forbid, eating ice cream or cake?) What emotions flash through your mind when they walk into your office?

It has been said that fat is the last bastion of permissible stereotyping and discrimination in our culture. It is no longer politically correct to make gay, lesbian, black, Jewish, Mexican, or transgender jokes, but we can still make fat jokes. Moreover, not a day goes by without reading or hearing about how bad being overweight or obese is, how it's going to kill us if we don't "win the war" against it. Do we as health care professionals really want to participate in demonizing fat and shaming people of higher weights—or do we want to help them care for their health?

According to recent research, "Bias and stigma are well-established barriers to improving public and personal health. Bias against people with obesity has been reported to have worsened as the prevalence of obesity has increased. These data suggest that the public increasingly understands that obesity is more than a simple problem of personal responsibility. But that understanding is not translating into improved social acceptance for people with higher weights. Social acceptance of people with obesity in education, employment, and family relations may be declining. That possibility is especially troubling in light of health effects associated with social isolation. Continued monitoring of public attitudes is essential to determine how these trends will evolve. Weight bias remains a significant source of harm to people living with obesity and a significant impediment to progress in reducing obesity's adverse effects."[7]

Could we all agree, then, that there is substantial fat prejudice in this country and that, if you grew up here or have spent a great deal of time living here, you probably have some bias against people of high weight, whether you are slim, normal weight, or are large-sized yourself? This is not a condemnation of your value system or integrity and does not make you a moral failure. It makes you someone who is, more or less, just like everyone else, in that we cannot help but absorb the covert and overt messages from the society we live in. The best we can do is to not turn away from recognizing and acknowledging our prejudices and biases, but to discover what they are and compassionately try to reverse them.

Will these prejudices and biases disappear completely? Who's to say? Probably not. But, because what we think consciously and, more to the point, unconsciously programs our feelings and behavior, it's far better to be aware of our biases so that we can modify them rather than walk around with blinders on. The alternative to self-knowledge is to roll merrily along, ignorant of what we think and unaware of why we're doing what we're doing. And in the case of medical professionals, it also means being part of the problem of treating patients of high weights rather than being part of the solution.

## ARE YOU SAYING THAT PEOPLE IN THE HEALTH PROFESSIONS HAVE BIASES AGAINST THE PATIENTS OF SIZE THAT THEY'RE TREATING?

This is what the research tells us. Although many doctors, nurses, and medical practitioners may not be strongly biased, many are. The attitudes run along a continuum as they do with nonmedical practitioners. You may be surprised about the results of research regarding health professionals and fat prejudice and stigmatization. "Even health care specialists have strong negative associations toward obese persons, indicating the pervasiveness of the stigma toward obesity. Notwithstanding, there appears to be a buffering factor, perhaps related to their experience in caring for obese patients, which reduces the bias."[8]

Doctors, in fact, may be nicer to "thin" patients than to "fat" patients. "A provocative new study suggests that they are—that thin patients are treated with more warmth and empathy than those who are overweight or obese. Doctors seemed just a bit nicer to their normal-weight patients, showing more empathy and warmth in their conversations. Although the study was relatively small, the findings are statistically significant. It's not like the physicians were being overtly negative or harsh," said the lead author, Dr. Kimberly A. Gudzune, an assistant professor of general internal medicine at the Johns Hopkins School of Medicine. "They were just not engaging patients in that rapport-building or making that emotional connection with the patient."[9] Yikes!

"For MDs who were underweight, normal weight and overweight we found strong explicit anti-fat bias."[10] Moreover, "doctors' and nurses' own weights may predict how helpful they are to patients with eating and weight concerns. Syntheses of the findings from the selected studies suggest that: normal-weight doctors and nurses were more likely than those who were overweight to use strategies to prevent obesity in patients, and also provide overweight or obese patients with general advice to achieve weight loss."[11] In fact, weight bias and stigma have compounded the problems of people whose weight falls outside of "normal" parameters. "Stigma and discrimination toward obese persons are pervasive and pose numerous consequences for their psychological and physical health. Despite decades of science documenting weight stigma, its public health implications are widely ignored. Instead, obese persons are blamed for their weight, with common perceptions that weight stigmatization is justifiable and may motivate individuals to adopt healthier behaviors. . . . On the basis of current findings, we propose that weight stigma is not a beneficial public health tool for reducing obesity. Rather, stigmatization of obese individuals threatens health, generates health disparities, and interferes with effective obesity intervention efforts."[12]

Moreover, people are not only blamed for their size or BMI or being out of shape but also held responsible for staying that way, as if they were given the choice to be slender but made a conscious decision to stay just as they are. Studies tell us that large people are rated "high on personal responsibility" for their weight and, consequently, were "disliked, evoked little pity and high anger, and received low ratings of helping tendencies."[13] Ouch!

---

Brain food for providers: Take a minute to examine your feelings about your patients of size. What are your honest reactions to treating them? Can you readily acknowledge any bias you have against them without judging yourself harshly? Do you feel angry at them or at yourself?

---

Unfortunately, "an accumulation of research has found that health care settings are a significant source of weight stigma, which undermines obese patients' opportunity to receive effective medical care. Both self-report and experimental research demonstrate negative stereotypes and attitudes toward obese patients by a range of health care providers and fitness professionals, including views that obese patients are lazy, lacking in self-discipline, dishonest, unintelligent, annoying, and noncompliant with treatment. There is also research indicating that providers spend less time in appointments and provide less health education with obese patients compared with thinner patients.

In response, obese individuals frequently report experiences of weight bias in health care. Obese patients also indicate that they feel disrespected by providers, perceive that they will not be taken seriously because of their weight, report that their weight is blamed for all of their medical problems, and are reluctant to address their weight concerns with providers."[14]

We understand that it is not your intent to treat higher-weight patients any differently than you do your thinner or normal-size patients. We get that, we really do. In fact, you may be the rare exception who attends to all your patients with equal kindness and compassion. But, even if this is the case, you probably have heard other doctors or health care professionals grousing about their "overweight" patients refusing to take responsibility for themselves, not caring about their health, or declining treatments like medication and surgeries that are designed to help them.

So, let's assume that many medical professionals have a bias against higher-weight patients. Of course, you might be thinking that there is one subgroup of medical providers who actually might be less judgmental and prejudiced against patients of size: practitioners themselves who have struggled or are struggling with eating and weight. Sadly, this is not generally the case, as they too have internalized the blame and shame of compulsive, emotional or mindless eating or simply have higher-than-average poundage due to genetics or other factors that put them on the heavier end of the weight spectrum.

### HOW EXACTLY DOES A HEALTH PROFESSIONALS' WEIGHT IMPACT TREATMENT OF HIGHER-WEIGHT OR EATING DYSREGULATED PATIENTS?

On top of your feelings about your own eating and size, your profession, unlike many others, can't help but shine a spotlight on the subject. There are a number of ways you may feel about your relationship with food and the scale and, whatever your mindset is, unless you are very conscientious and careful, it will affect how you feel about and treat your patients.

Later in this chapter, we'll be talking about options for handling your emotions, reactions, and resultant provider-patient dynamics. For now, as you go through the possibilities below, simply notice how you feel reading them, especially any discomfort which arises. If that happens, just note it and stay with it until you feel compassion for yourself rather than judgment. You are human and allowed to have the same foibles and emotions as the rest of us.

If you are going to try to treat your patients with compassion rather than judgment, this is a good time to start understanding your feelings about your own eating struggles.

Here are eight possibilities and how they may cause you to react to patients with eating concerns or high weights:

1. *Situation*: You may be vigilant about eating healthfully, exercising, and keeping a watchful eye on the scale, believing that if you can do this, your patients can too.
   *Reaction*: bafflement, disgust, contempt, or frustration

2. *Situation*: You may struggle against mindless eating, skipping out on the gym, or going for a run, and feel an unwelcome, uneasy kinship with your patients who share your battle fatigue.
   *Reaction*: guilt, shame, vulnerability, or hopelessness

3. *Situation*: You may, as a naturally thin person blessed with a fast metabolism, expect others to eat what they want as you do without packing on pounds.
   *Reaction*: bafflement, disbelief, contempt, or pity

4. *Situation*: You may, as a former person with eating difficulties who has been able to shed pounds and keep them off, be unable to fathom why other people can't stop eating when they're full or pass up sweets and treats as you have learned to do.
   *Reaction*: bafflement, contempt, disgust, or frustration

5. *Situation*: You long ago may have given up on trying to eradicate mindless eating, leaving you unable to imagine ever again being motivated to try to improve your eating habits.
   *Reaction*: guilt, shame, vulnerability, or hopelessness

6. *Situation*: You may refuse to acknowledge that your eating habits are poor and that you're not the fit triathlon competitor you were in college, yet find yourself ducking doctors' visits and lab work alike, except in the most dire medical circumstances.
   *Reaction*: discomfort, shame, evasiveness, or guilt

7. *Situation*: You may feel caught in the spotlight as a role model regarding weight and fitness and see no reason that your size should complicate or compromise treating patients—whatever their size.
   *Reaction*: annoyance, uneasiness, or rebelliousness

8. *Situation*: You may be so uncomfortable with your own size or state of physical fitness that you wouldn't dream of bringing up the subject of a patient's
eating or BMI, lest the conversation reflect badly on you as a health care
role model.
*Reaction*: anxiety, vulnerability

---

Brain food for providers: Do you have compassion for yourself if you
have eating or weight struggles? What would make you afraid to feel
self-compassion? What emotions have you felt toward your high-weight
patients, how did they get expressed, and how did patients react? What
can you do to manage your own self-talk and reactions better in the future?

---

Let's consider how the above situations and reactions might play out in
your office while treating patients. The most likely interpersonal dynamics
that could occur in this situation between you and your patients include
denial, personalizing, overidentification, intellectualization, projection, and
displacement.

### Denial

You may be so uncomfortable about your own size that it affects whether
and how you discuss patients' eating problems or discomfort with their weight.
You may be in such denial about your own eating problems that you ignore
the needs of your patients, leading you to do a less than effective job in helping
them with similar issues. They may ask, "Hey, doc, can you help me with my
overeating?" (actually, they'll probably ask you to help them with their weight,
since many patients will not acknowledge that, often, weight problems may
actually be eating problems), and you may say, "Watch your portions," and
simply move on to another subject.

### Personalizing

Especially if your patients come in complaining about the same health
problems visit after visit, you may take it as a personal affront that they're not
listening to you and, therefore, react with anger. You might think, "They're just
wasting my time." Because they're failing to reach their goals or, worse, not

even attempting to do so, you may believe that they're blaming you, as if to say, "Doc, what's wrong with *you* that you can't help *me*?"

### Overidentification

When you overidentify with patients who are struggling with similar eating or weight issues, you may lose perspective, feel as helpless as they do, and forget that your job is to help them get beyond their sense of powerlessness. When you overidentify, you lose your power to heal your patients.

### Intellectualization

You are intellectualizing, moving from heart to head mode, when you tell patients, "Just eat smaller portions" or "Don't go out to eat so much." When this happens, you miss the chance to connect with how patients are feeling about their eating problems, which is often more important to them than your advice. Instead, hone your skill in empathy reflection, a remarkably effective tool for establishing trust and rapport, and for letting your patient know that he or she has been heard. We'll discuss this helpful relational tool further in Chapter 8.

### Projection

In its simplest terms for our purpose here, projection occurs when something about us makes us so uncomfortable that we can't see it in ourselves but readily see it in others. A tightwad may never fail to point out other cheapskates, an irate person may insist she's not angry and, instead, blame others for having a bad temper, and a person who feels frightened or helpless may berate someone else for not having gumption or being proactive.

You may become frustrated with patients who have the same difficulties as you have: Why can't you/they ever say no to sweets, exercise regularly, and think about the health consequences of your/their food choices. Rather than acknowledging having shame about these behaviors and offering them compassion, you might scold your patient for having them by admonishing, "You're never going to get your cholesterol under control if you don't stop eating the way you do." How much easier to focus on the problem in your patient than in yourself.

### Displacement

When we displace feelings, we project them in a safe direction away from ourselves in order to release the tension that's been building up in us because of them. If you are frustrated with patients who you believe aren't taking care of themselves and are careful not to show your frustration, you might instead get annoyed at your generally conscientious nurse when he forgets to give you the chart for your next patient. And he may wonder whatever has gotten into you.

---

Brain food for providers: Which of the above types of interactions do you recognize having had with patients? Are any of them frequent or common? What can you do to make sure these interactions don't happen?

---

## DO MY PATIENTS ACTUALLY VIEW ME AS MORE OR LESS EFFECTIVE DEPENDING ON MY WEIGHT?

We'd like to say it isn't so, but, the answer is yes. "Researchers identify that the widely identified weight bias or stigma extends into the exam room. Patients of an overweight or obese physician were less trusting of their doctors, less likely to take the physicians' lifestyle advice, and more likely to switch to a different doctor. Key factors suggested as contributors to a physician being overweight or obese included a lack of work-life balance and poor sleep habits."[15] With half of doctors and well over half of nurses being overweight or obese, this is just one more barrier (albeit one that being aware of bias and overcoming it can change) to patients of size receiving effective care and treatment for their eating and weight concerns.[16]

We now see that bias can come from both directions and that neither professional nor patient can easily avoid it. The subject is complex. Higher weight may be seen as a character flaw in doctors, which sometimes makes patients uneasy, especially if they are also heavy. Patients may believe that if a doctor cannot help herself, she won't be able to help them—which is not necessarily the case. Moreover, while some "patients are more apt to trust overweight doctors when it comes to diet advice, they're also more likely to feel that the overweight doctor is judging them about their weight."[17] This is likely a case of projection, as described earlier. To complicate matters, one study found that "overweight doctors are actually less likely to address a patient's weight issues, and feel less confident in counseling about diet and exercise."[18] Because patients are judging doctors and doctors are judging patients, everybody loses out.

What does that mean for medical practice and, specifically, for practitioners? That health care providers who struggle with overeating or weight concerns should give up and find another way to make a living? Of course not. It means that they, too, need to abandon dieting, stop focusing exclusively on weight, and learn how the psychology of eating can help them reach their eating and health goals. As Margaret McCartney, a general practitioner from Glasgow, Scotland, says, "We should not assume that fat doctors are bad doctors or are 'not thinking about it.' Those of us who have gained, lost, gained, lost, and gained weight again are only too aware of our failings. The medical profession should be tolerant of these—the same problems that our other patients face."[19] Amen.

## I WANT TO TREAT MY HIGHER-WEIGHT PATIENTS BETTER THAN I HAVE BEEN DOING, SO WHERE DO I BEGIN?

You begin with yourself. By putting your work and your role in it into perspective. As American author and historian Edward Everett Hale said, "I am only one, but I am one. I cannot do everything, but I can do something. And because I cannot do everything, I will not refuse to do the something that I can do."[20] It's true, you don't have the time or knowledge to do a full court press to change your patients' eating or exercise or body-shaming habits. We appreciate that your window of opportunity for this subject in a typical 15-minute office visit is likely to be one or two minutes at most.

So, what can you do, especially on the psychological front? For starters, you can recognize that, as with every other condition you've ever encountered or treated, sometimes you will succeed in a cure and sometimes you won't. You can remind yourself that you may do your utmost and still not produce the outcome you (or your patient) desire. You can be aware that you have your limits and that patients have theirs. There, doesn't that feel better already?

However, here are eight simple, direct actions you can take that will strongly (and perhaps surprisingly) influence your patients' ability to make progressive changes in the eating and health arenas.

### Nix the rescue fantasy

It will help enormously if you opt out of being a part of patients' rescue fantasies, the ones in which you do all the heavy lifting and they do little or none of it. It's crucial to understand that they may feverishly project this desire to be rescued (a.k.a. save me from myself) onto you, but that you must resist because it's a set-up for you and them to fail. Here's why: If you succeed in rescuing them and they eat better and become more fit because you've stayed on them like a Marine drill sergeant and they've changed only to please you, they've learned nothing about themselves and will almost certainly regress to old, unhealthy behaviors without your ongoing reinforcement. Remember, they can't carry you around in their pocket like a phone app.

Alternately, if they don't succeed when you've bent over backward to help them, who do you think they're going to blame? You, very possibly. So nix the rescue fantasy. For sure, collaborate and cooperate to get the job done, possibly by suggesting small steps and strategies to generate consistency in wellness-promoting behaviors. Then remember that you are doing your best and your patients are doing theirs. It may be difficult to give up the rescue fantasy (psychotherapists battle against it regularly), but give it up you must if you want your patients to succeed.

### Treat patients with respect

Respect does not mean always agreeing with patients, but it does involve taking their perspectives (ridiculous or unhealthy as they sound and may indeed be) seriously. If they say that they're too busy to get to a gym, don't tell them that's not so because you're the busiest guy in your practice and still manage to get up at 4:30 every morning to work out. Respect means acknowledging that they *believe* they have good reasons for doing what they're doing, or not doing what you wish (or even) they wish they were doing. Having respect comes from the place in you that says you haven't lived their lives, but if you had, you might be acting the same way they are.

Being respectful includes never shaming, ridiculing, or stigmatizing patients for their lack of progress with food or fitness. Never, not once, no matter how frustrated and helpless you feel. You may not be pleased that they are unhealthy or you may worry that they're at risk for serious and fatal diseases. You may not care for their cavalier, blasé, or defensive attitudes about their bodies or their health. But, to be effective, you will need to put aside your feelings and take a more strategic approach. The truth is that you don't need to approve of how your patients take care of themselves in order to help them make progress. What is essential is for you to start from a place of respect and empathy, no matter how exasperated you feel. Over time respect builds trust and makes patients more likely to speak up when they are finally ready to consider or attempt change.

### Exude empathy

Failing to express empathy will likely derail a constructive relationship with patients of higher weights. "While BMI was not associated with perception of physician empathy, higher frequency of weight stigmatizing situations was negatively associated with perception of physician empathy. Reducing weight stigma in primary care could improve doctor-patient relationships and quality of care in patients with obesity."[21]

The way you treat patients respectfully is by empathizing with them. This means trying to understand and validate their experience and take a walk in their shoes by listening closely to their explanations (or excuses) and by using empathy reflections which is a way of responding to patients in such a way that they have no doubt that you "get" what they're thinking, saying, or feeling. This basic, learnable skill will improve your relationship with your patients exponentially. Just as a patient will not hear anything you say about the lump on her knee until you tell her that it is not cancer, a patient struggling with challenging eating is unlikely to trust you with the real truth until it is evident that you are coming from a place of caring and understanding. You'll learn more about empathic reflection in Chapter 8.

### Lead with compassion

Compassion does not mean agreeing with what patients say or do, seeing things the same way, approving of their actions, or even liking them very much. Compassion is a cousin to empathy and involves being kind to others who are hurting or suffering, understanding that they're human and have frailties and limits, and connecting to them by knowing that they're striving to improve in spite of their flaws. Said simply, it's one part forgiveness of their imperfections and one part wanting to relieve their suffering. Really, is that so hard?

Compassion is the opposite of being hard on someone or yourself. Here are some examples. Rather than be angry at a colleague who misdiagnosed a patient and left you stuck cleaning up his mess, you feel compassion that your colleague did the best she could under egregious circumstances. Or instead of feeling contemptuous of a patient who can't avoid fast food for more than a week, recognizing that he is doing the best he can right now and that coming down hard on him isn't going to make getting healthier any easier. Remember, too, that by making improvements in lifestyle choices, our best can always get better.

Many doctors and health care professionals are tough on themselves and show little, if any, self-compassion. They fear not riding themselves hard, letting themselves off the hook, and forgiving themselves for being human. If you are this kind of provider, you might find it difficult to not come down hard on patients and to show them compassion. That's because you don't have much for yourself. In that case, this is a necessary skill for you to learn to apply both to yourself and to your patients. As you learn to be more compassionate toward higher-weight patients, you'll find, surprisingly, that this attitude may carry over into how you treat yourself. And as you become kinder to yourself, compassion will become more the norm in how you respond to your patients.

A reminder that being compassionate does not mean giving people a free pass all the time. Nor does it mean that you don't expect patients to make efforts on their behalf and be accountable for their own wellness. It means being kind when they fail and letting them know that you still care about and value them. When you lead with compassion, you're putting your best therapeutic foot forward and making clients feel less badly about themselves. When we're critical, we make people feel badly about themselves which kills motivation. Alternately, when we're compassionate, they feel better about themselves which helps motivate them to do better.

One of the biggest obstacles to progress that psychotherapists treating clients with eating and weight concerns come across is clients' pronounced lack of compassion for themselves. Briefly, here are five myths about self-compassion. It (1) is a form of self-pity; (2) means weakness; (3) will make people complacent; (4) is narcissistic; and (5) is selfish.[22] Actually, self-compassion means nothing more or less than feeling badly about someone's suffering and in this case, that someone is you. Empirical evidence suggests that self-compassion can actually help reduce shame, improve body image and eating behavior.[23] A free clinical intervention, with positive side effects!

### Listen actively

Another skill that psychotherapists employ which is a bonus in every professional and personal situation is active listening, which involves setting aside everything you want to say and putting 100 percent of your attention on what another person is saying. This means listening to words as well as attending to tone and body language, while simultaneously keeping an internal focus on seeking understanding of what is being said. The aim is to tune into and comprehend what the other person means—that is, their intent—not merely to understand the words they're saying.

You want to be constantly translating words, tone, affect, and body language into meaning and continuously thinking, "What is she really saying? What am I supposed to be understanding from what is being said? What is she trying to tell me?" If a patient maintains eye contact with you, slightly increases inflection, smiles, and sits up straighter when she says she can't wait to join the gym, that's one message. If a patient makes the same statement and simultaneously breaks eye contact and crosses her arms in front of her, there's quite another story being told.

### Collaborate on setting realistic goals

No matter what kind of practitioners we are, sometimes we just get caught up in the joy of seeing patients succeed. We're happy for them that they're training for a marathon or have begun working with a registered dietician or a diabetes educator. We definitely want to encourage them and let them know we're in their corner. However, sometimes—and this is yet another lesson that psychotherapists learn early on—we end up working harder than our patients, and that's because we have gone overboard in setting unrealistic goals for them.

Yes, there are many patients who train for and run a marathon who continue to run regularly long after the event is over. However, there are probably as many, if not more, who train their hearts out and exhaust their bodies, finish the marathon, and never lace up their running shoes again. Often, patients who are unhappy with their weight overreach and think they can do more than is realistically possible, setting themselves up for injury and long-term failure. They may resent when you try to scale down their goals and talk to them about baby steps, but that is what you must do if you want them to continue to make progress. Too many patients have underlying all-or-nothing thinking, which turns on for something, then later turns off. So be careful with your own enthusiasm and make sure that patients' eating and exercise goals seem both achievable and sustainable for them.

### Think like a shrink

Think like a shrink, which means using as much as you know about psychology—particularly the psychology of eating—to help heal your patients. If they seem depressed, feel free to ask if something is going on in their lives that might be stressing or distressing them. You may find out that the woman who keeps complaining that she can't stop night eating just lost her husband and is turning to food for comfort. Or you may discover that a gay or lesbian late adolescent is being bullied at college and drives through the fast-food window every night before returning to his or her dorm room. When there's a change in behavior from healthy to unhealthy, you will always want to ask yourself, "Why now?" This is what psychotherapists are taught to do and it is an invaluable question to ask whenever there are shifts in behavior in a negative direction.

Psychotherapists know that behavioral motivation is rarely unilateral. There's almost always an upside and a downside. So when they're presented with the upside from patients who say, for example, "I haven't watched TV and eaten a pint of ice cream in one sitting all week," psychotherapists automatically wonder if there's a downside and might ask, "Is that easy or difficult for you? Is there any self-talk going on in your mind that might sabotage this healthy new behavior?" Equally, when they're presented with a downside such as, "I can't stop watching TV without eating a pint of ice cream every night," psychotherapists assume there might be a brighter side to the story and ask, "Is there anything that would help you stop this behavior? What does the voice in you that wants to take care of yourself say about eating ice cream watching TV every night?"

Asking these types of questions to root out internal conflict is an important psychological tool that gets patients thinking and can help them begin to anticipate obstacles and formulate a plan to regulate behavior. Even if you cannot solve their problems for them, you always can get the ball rolling by asking great questions that make them curious to explore their own beliefs and emotions. It is in that internal investigation, rather than in your well-intentioned admonitions to improve their behaviors, that crucial answers will be found. Health and wellness coaches are taught that behavioral change is more likely to last when a person is able to find his or her own solutions that motivate from within.

One more thing that psychotherapists know and recognize in the patient-provider relationship is that transference and countertransference will occur.[24]

Without getting too clinical, think of transference as patients viewing and reacting to providers as if they were major, significant people in their past or present—for example, if you come off as authoritarian and they had a my-way-or-the-highway kind of mother, they may either rebel against you or go all passive and yes you to death. Or, if you tend to be a "just the facts kind of clinician," and they have a similar kind of unemotional, detached father or husband, your lack of warm and fuzzy may trigger resentment and anger.

To complicate matters, not only do patients have transference toward us, we may have what's called countertransference toward them—a whiny patient may unconsciously remind you of your constant complainer of a father or spouse, a patient whom you believe to be depressed may laugh off your suggestion that he is and trigger feelings about your depressed sister who would never admit the depths of her despair and eventually committed suicide. Being mindful of this consideration will help us maintain professional equanimity and empathy with all of our patients.

---

Brain food for providers: What strategies will be most helpful for improving your relationship with higher-weight patients? Which strategies will come most easily for you? Which ones will be harder to adopt? What benefit would you and your patients derive from learning to practice these strategies until they are more natural to you?

---

We want to repeat that we're not expecting you to morph into psychotherapists. You have your very essential niche and they have theirs. But, just as medicine has changed psychotherapy for the better—making it more evidence based and using medical technology to understand the brain and emotions, for example—the psychology of eating has much to teach doctors and health care professionals to improve their care of themselves and their patients.

Providers, try . . .

1. Telling yourself that despite whatever eating and weight concerns you may have, you can still help your patients.
2. Talking with colleagues about how to manage fat bias and weight prejudice in the office.

3. Examining and changing the beliefs you have that generate fat bias and weight prejudice.

4. Allowing yourself to feel frustrated with your own and your patients' struggles with food and the scale.

5. Striving to understand the dynamics at play with you and your higher-weight patients, including projection, denial, intellectualizing, personalizing, displacement, and overidentification.

6. Leading with compassion and empathy when treating patients with eating and weight concerns, understanding that even though you may not do it perfectly, these tools promote patient progress and success in improving lifestyle behaviors.

7. If you are interested, reading books on the basic elements of psychotherapy such as Sheldon Roth, M.D.'s *Psychotherapy: The Art of Wooing Nature* and Leston Havens, M.D.'s *A Safe Place: A Glimpse Into the Private World and Complex Relationship of Patient and Therapist*.

8. Learning more about the psychology of eating and about how to resolve your own eating problems, if they exist. (See our resource list at the end of this book.)

9. Gently making compassionate but corrective comments when others express size or weight stigmatizing remarks and establishing a zero tolerance policy for that kind of talk in the office.

Patients, try . . .

1. Gently educating health professionals about how to best approach your eating or weight concerns.

2. Speaking up assertively and appropriately if you feel judged or stigmatized about your weight or size.

3. Not putting on a happy face about it when you feel shamed or invalidated by your health care provider.

4. Not dieting and instead looking to becoming a "normal," nutritious eater by finding an eating disorders therapist or appropriately trained eating coach to help you.

5. Making sure your doctor takes a weight, dieting, and an eating history for you, noting how often you've lost weight and regained it.

6. Letting providers know what they do or say that works for you and what doesn't.
7. Not judging your providers by their size, but giving them the benefit of the doubt that they can be of help to you, until proven otherwise.

# 7

# Strategies to Help Patients Achieve Their Eating and Health Goals

## (I Get It—We're Talking Health Gains, Not Weight Loss!)

- The current state and failure of medical practice regarding outcomes such as weight and BMI and the need to refine our focus on health promotion and controllable lifestyle behaviors
- The argument for helping patients develop a psychological foundation for sustainable improvements in thinking and behavior regarding food, fitness, and wellness success
- The "wellness skill set" that patients can learn to sustain health-promoting behaviors

Right about now you might be relieved to know that diets have failed patients and not the other way around, and you also might be feeling a bit uneasy about having recommended calorie restriction to your patients in the past, albeit with the best of intentions. Moreover, you might be puzzled about the most effective approach to help patients attain—and maintain—their eating and fitness goals. After all, they look to you to provide information and strategies to guide them toward improved health. One point you might consider is that many patients actually have been succeeding at weight loss—but over and over and over again.

As health care providers, most of us were trained to define weight loss as the single most important outcome for our higher-weight patients. In medicine, we typically evaluate success in terms of health-related outcome parameters, and since the invention of the scale, a patient's weight has always been the major part of the equation. In addition to weight, health status has been measured by BMI, which takes into account patients' weight for their height in determining whether they are "underweight," "normal weight," "overweight," or "obese." Weight goals are so ingrained in our medical culture that we rarely question whether they represent a true measure of wellness for the patient. This sad reality is likely to be the case regardless of our health care discipline.

---

Brain food for providers: What do you find helpful about using patients' weights to measure their health? What do you not find helpful? What other measures would you consider as equally, or more, important when evaluating overall wellness?

---

Brain food for patients: What would you like your doctors and health care providers to attend to and assess when determining your health other than weight loss? How do you feel when they overfocus on weight or BMI as a measure of wellness?

---

## WEIGHT OR BMI ALONE IS AN INADEQUATE INDICATOR OF HEALTH

In assessing a patient's level of wellness, there are several problems with relying on the number on the scale or on quantitative outcomes alone. First, weight and BMI may be useful for research purposes and convenient for tracking progress, but in a vacuum, "they are meaningless in determining someone's *health* status."[1] Additionally, focusing on weight or BMI in lieu of other markers of health and well-being has unintended consequences in terms of causing patients to overfocus on them at the expense of other measures, including level of fitness, which research demonstrates is a better indicator of health.[2] This overfocus breeds fear, stigma, and shame that can lead patients to give up on improving health-promoting behaviors altogether if they fail to achieve or maintain weight loss.

Moreover, weight loss, by itself, does not necessarily improve health, as evidenced by people who lose weight due to illness, anorexia, or depression, for example. A normal or low BMI may not indicate a healthy or lean body, because BMI tells us nothing about a given individual's health habits, percentage of lean body mass or where fat is stored in the body. In fact, the medical literature suggests that even people of normal or low weight may have metabolic dysfunction and increased cardiovascular risk related to a relative excess of visceral fat stores[3, 4] resulting from such diverse factors as genetics, sedentary lifestyle, weight cycling, stress, hormonal factors, or an over-processed, low nutrient-density diet. Metabolic dysfunction related to excessive visceral fat stores can put patients at increased risk for cardiovascular disease, type 2 diabetes, and certain cancers, regardless of their BMI.[5]

Conversely, according to Dr. Carl Lavie, author of *The Obesity Paradox*, "When people start to develop exercise habits that improve their cardio fitness and muscle strength, everything else improves (i.e. body composition, overall health profile, risk for disease and death)."[6] According to Dr. Lavie, "exercise and fitness can clearly protect you from death and disease regardless of weight."[7] The point is that thinness, BMI, and even lab values *in and of themselves* do not provide a complete or meaningful picture of either physical or psychological well-being, satisfaction, or happiness. We would do better to focus on lifestyle habits that actually do improve health, such as nutritious eating habits, consistent exercise, avoidance of smoking, stress management, adequate sleep, relational connection, and life balance. This attention to controllable lifestyle factors represents a major focus of Lifestyle Medicine, which we will discuss further in Chapter 8.

## WHAT IS WEIGHT CYCLING AND WHAT ARE ITS DANGERS?

As discussed in Chapter 3, research indicates that weight loss in our society is likely to be temporary, because most people regain most or all of the weight they lose, only to start the process anew. Thus, the number on the scale on any given day does not necessarily represent the full measure of lasting success—or health—for the patient. Temporary behavioral change leads to temporary results, and external motivators rarely work as well as internal ones when permanent behavioral change is the goal. As we know from experience, lost weight will generally return when the diet or illness or other proximate cause ends, and many dieters lose and gain weight over and over again, a process known as "yo-yo dieting," or weight cycling.

In her book, *Health at Every Size*, Linda Bacon, Ph.D., cites a study by Dulloo et al. that reports that weight fluctuation is an "independent risk factor for metabolic disease," including diabetes, hypertension, and cardiovascular diseases, independent of body weight.[8] According to research scientist and psychology professor Tracy Mann, Ph.D., an expert on the psychology of eating, dieting, and self-control, and the author of *Secrets from the Eating Lab*, a growing body of evidence suggests that weight cycling actually contributes to metabolic harm for the long term and may be more dangerous than maintaining a stable weight at the higher end of the weight or BMI recommendations: "The majority of the evidence suggests that weight cycling is associated with an increased risk of illness and death. Those studies find that you are better off maintaining a stable obese weight than starting obese, losing weight, and gaining it back."[9]

From the literature and conclusions reviewed in Chapter 3, it would seem that a more appropriate wellness-promoting goal would be the *avoidance of weight cycling* by helping our patients achieve lasting, rather than temporary, *behavioral* change, since behaviors implemented consistently become habits and are more likely to stick.

## LASTING BEHAVIORAL CHANGE REQUIRES A SOLID PSYCHOLOGICAL FOUNDATION AND SKILL SET

We know that permanent behavior change is not simply a question of motivation, and that, as Jennifer Taitz, Psy.D., author of *End Emotional Eating*, puts it, willpower "is less about will than it is about skill."[10] Rather, we need to help our patients recognize that lasting success in maintaining wellness-promoting attitudes (such as body appreciation) and lifestyle behaviors (such as "normal" eating, regular physical activity, effective stress management, adequate sleep, and maintaining healthy relationships) lies in mastering certain foundational beliefs, thoughts, attitudes, and learnable life skills that are actually effective in improving self-efficacy and thus driving permanent behavior change. You might be surprised to know that *these foundational contributors to successful long-term behavior change are psychological in nature* and include identifying and regulating emotions that trigger mindless and non-nutritious eating. Also important are skills related to mindful attention, self-acceptance, and autonomous motivation, as described by Beth Frates, M.D., and Margaret Moore, M.B.A., in the *Lifestyle Medicine* textbook chapter titled "Health and Wellness Coaching Skills for Lasting Change."[11] We put the cart before the horse when we encourage patients to white-knuckle nutritious eating and weight-related behaviors before they have the attitudes and skills to forge those behaviors into habits that sustain desirable outcomes.

The foundational beliefs, thoughts, attitudes, and life skills that characterize psychological well-being cannot be measured the same way that weight or lab values can, but they play an absolutely critical role in assuring lasting success for individuals who seek to achieve permanent wellness-promoting behavior change. They are fundamental tenets of the psychology of success, and, for the patient, they amount to nothing less than the deliberate, incremental creation of a new self-concept.[12] It is this self-concept, coupled with a deeply entrenched internal locus of control and effective self-regulation strategies, that can motivate patients to commit to the consistent and sustainable thoughts and attitudes that drive wellness-related behaviors. Alas, we have been trying (to little avail) to heal our patients from the outside in rather than from the inside out!

It is important to understand that mastering the beliefs, feelings/emotions, self-talk, and attitudes that facilitate consistent wellness-promoting behaviors ultimately leads to improvements in health and wellness, with or without weight loss. Without a psychological foundation of self-efficacy and self-regulation in place, the behaviors we recommend and the outcomes we seek for our patients risk being unsustainable, like a huge house without a solid foundation. Once these foundational components are in place, however, lasting change is patient-motivated, patient-driven, and far more likely to be achieved and sustained for the long term.

---

Brain food for providers and patients: What life skills do you believe are essential to engage in good health care, especially around eating and weight concerns?

---

## THE WELLNESS SKILL SET CAN BE LEARNED AND PRACTICED
## TO IMPROVE BEHAVIORS AND OUTCOMES

Please don't let this new concept of a Wellness Skill Set scare you. You chose this book to learn a new way to benefit your patients. Success for them hinges, quite simply, on identifying and improving the conscious and subconscious set of beliefs that drive their eating, exercise, and other self-care behaviors. It also rests on the development of important life skills (including self-regulation) that improve our patients' chances of implementing and sustaining those wellness behaviors over a lifetime. Once these life skills are learned, the patient benefits from enhanced awareness of and conscious attunement to internal sensations, cues, emotions, and needs, as well as a nonjudgmental, conscious appreciation of their values, strengths, and challenges.

People who have developed this skill set improve their ability to visualize their desired outcome and set and reach appropriate goals through planning, focus, consistency, and persistence. These competencies contribute to the development of enhanced self-efficacy and the generation of a positive self-concept, which may have been missing in the patient's life, whether or not he or she realized it. With this awareness, an internal locus of control, and with deliberately chosen constructive beliefs, attitudes, and life skills in place, our patients will be better able to implement wellness-enhancing thoughts, as well as provider-recommended behaviors and actions, consistently, rather than engaging in the on-again, off-again dieting behavior that leads to stagnation and weight cycling.

## IF NOT WEIGHT AND BMI, THEN WHAT PATIENT ATTRIBUTES DO INDICATE SUCCESS?

So what does success look like for the (formerly) dysregulated and now "normal" eater? On the surface, we may notice that these successful people maintain a comfortable weight, eat healthfully, exercise regularly, manage stress well, and have stable, mutually satisfying relationships. But what is truly foundational for them are the qualities that we cannot see. When it comes to the aspects of wellness that patients can control (outside of genetics, injury or illness, for example), successful people have eight common psychological attributes that are key to resolving dysregulated eating.

These successful people are (1) self-regulated, (2) self-compassionate, (3) attuned (to their strengths as well as to their appetites), (4) clear visualizers, (5) process oriented, (6) positive, (7) persistent (high frustration tolerance with the ability to delay gratification), and (8) consistent. The good news for those of us who were not born with temperaments which might lead us in these directions, or who have lost any innate predisposition to be this way, is that these attributes can be deliberately adopted, learned, practiced, and integrated into one's life. Many of our patients are not even aware that they lack these attributes. Once they decide to adopt them, however, they are on the road to developing an internal locus of control and the power and self-efficacy that comes with it. Furthermore, these traits are interrelated, such that progress in one area can actually promote progress in the others, facilitating rapid growth and success.

### Self-regulation

Most doctors and nonmental health care providers likely have never given much thought to this vitally important attribute of those who succeed at maintaining wellness-enhancing behaviors over the long haul. Albert Bandura, Ph.D., father of Social Cognitive Theory of human behavior, describes self-regulation as including "self monitoring of one's behavior, it's determinants, and its effects; judgment of one's behavior in relation to personal standards and environmental circumstances, and affective self-reaction," and as "provid[ing] the very basis for purposeful action."[13] Bandura notes that self-regulation is closely tied to self-efficacy, which he defines as "people's beliefs about their capabilities to exercise control over their own level of functioning and over events that affect their lives," and he adds, "People's beliefs in their efficacy influence the choices they make, their aspirations, how much effort they mobilize in a given endeavor, [and] how long they persevere."[14]

The ability to self-regulate is thus important to sustaining motivation as well as behavior, and many dysregulated eaters, due to the personality traits discussed in Chapter 4, including all-or-nothing thinking and tendencies toward perfectionism, are weak in this area. Moreover, many dysregulated eaters have self-regulation problems beyond their struggles with food. Consider a person who habitually stays late at the office in order to complete important projects, despite the fact that he or she is exhausted. Or the individual who alternates between TV binges and giving up TV for months at a time. Or folks who regularly ignore their internal signals and overdo exercise at the gym, then chronically suffer from soreness or injury that impedes their progress toward sustainable fitness.

It probably won't surprise you to consider how these types of self-regulation problems affect many chronic dieters who are also high achievers. In order to excel and please others, many of us override our own feelings, needs, and desires for the good of the project, group, or organization. This makes us successful in our professional lives, for example, but may lead to physical and emotional depletion over time, increasing our risk of seeking solace through eating.

Effective self-regulation involves an individual sensing and identifying internal affective states (such as emotions and moods), recognizing dysregulation, and making corrections to move into greater balance. Skilled self-regulation (defined behaviorally as "the ability to act in your long-term best interest, consistent with your deepest values" and emotionally as "the ability to calm yourself down when you're upset and cheer yourself up when you're down")[15] is about maintaining life balance and adequate levels of emotional energy through intentional self-care not only when obstacles arise but even when things are going well, before you "need it."

It includes planning ahead, commitment to preventive and ongoing self-care, self-attunement (not just to food but also to the need for rest, stimulation, companionship, nurturing, play, and self-expression), and ongoing attention to our mind-body-behavior connection. Self-regulation is rooted in awareness and self-attunement, acceptance of what you are experiencing in the moment, recognizing what you value, and making a commitment to acting in your own best interest, regardless of circumstances or events. It is thus, emotionally speaking, about designing your vision for your life deliberately and then *responding*, rather than *reacting*, to the vagaries of daily life, while each day making choices in accordance with your deepest values.

Jennifer Taitz, Psy.D., describes research indicating that people who binge eat struggle with skills related to emotional intelligence and emotion regulation: "Research finds that difficulty in identifying and understanding emotions, as well as problems regulating them, influences binge eating more than gender, food restriction, or overvaluing shape and weight do (Whiteside et al., 2007)."[16] Taitz explains the importance of and interrelationship among awareness, emotional intelligence, and self-regulation in understanding dysregulated eating beautifully in her book, *End Emotional Eating*, which we highly recommend to providers and patients. In her chapter on mindfulness, she reminds us, "If you are in the habit of eating to stop feeling, you may confuse emotional pain with hunger . . . eating may serve as a way to avoid or escape emotions. When you bring awareness to your emotions, you may choose how to respond, rather than habitually reacting."[17]

As you have learned in earlier chapters, many dysregulated eaters have weak self-regulation skills. They may skip breakfast because they have "more important" things to do, or sleep through their alarm clock after having stayed up too late the night before, and wind up hungry and depleted mid-morning when they encounter a plate of cream-filled donuts in the break room. Starving, they may down two of them, then binge at lunch an hour later because they believe they've already ruined the day by impulsively having eaten foods that are "bad" for them. This is in important and often overlooked reason that many motivated high achievers struggle with their weight. Their all-or-nothing thinking and overfocus on work over play that enhances their success in the outside world robs them of their attunement to their inner signals of hunger, satiety, anxiety, and frustration. When they become depleted, often because of lack of awareness and planning (due to focusing on what seem to them "more pressing things"), they react by trying to refuel with whatever food is available. They then react to that behavior with punishing, critical self-talk, generating a self-destructive vicious cycle.

At this point, you have likely figured out that successful self-regulation is intimately tied not only to keeping a clear vision in mind in order to execute it but also to maintaining effective self-care during the process of working toward goals. What types of thoughts and activities constitute effective self-care? Are we referring to the massages, shopping excursions, or mani-pedis that are the stuff of high self-esteem and indulgent self-care in media images and magazines? Hardly. According to Karen R. Koenig's earlier works, *Nice Girls Finish Fat* and *Starting Monday*, stellar self-care includes such activities as setting appropriate boundaries with others, engaging in constructive, positive, and supportive self-talk, learning to be aware of, identify, and take responsibility for your feelings (a concept known as emotional intelligence),[18] learning to meet the needs behind those feelings in constructive ways (rather than with food, alcohol, drugs, emotional freak-outs, or melt downs), keeping yourself intellectually challenged, getting timely medical checkups, planning ahead for sustenance and pleasure as well as for deadlines, and setting aside time to relax, sleep, play, dream, create, or do nothing.

The deliberate prioritization of life balance through the practice of excellent self-care enables patients to avoid becoming emotionally depleted and losing their motivation to persist in striving toward their goals when the going gets tough. Moreover, good self-care, when internalized as a habit, sends a message to the subconscious that one is deserving and worthy of kindness, nurturing, and support (sound like self-compassion, anyone?), and this attitude of wor-thiness and deservedness provides the foundation for ongoing, consistent commitment to thinking and acting in one's own best interest. This habitual commitment to self-care and self-regulation results in increased self-efficacy and personal success in many areas of life, not only in health and wellness.

In his best-selling book, *Goals! How to Get Everything Your Want—Faster Than You Ever Thought Possible*, expert management consultant, trainer, and speaker Brian Tracy refers to this habit of clarifying values, planning ahead, and working on the plan consistency and in a regulated fashion as key to suc-cess in business.[19] These success strategies, not traditionally part of medical education, can teach us a great deal about how to help patients sustain moti-vation. Tracy outlines his seven-step method for goal attainment in his book *Change Your Thinking, Change Your Life*. The steps include "decid[ing] exactly what you want" (understanding that the simple process of defining your goals makes it easier to prioritize your time well), writing down goals (which helps to clarify them and increase resolve), being willing to "pay the price" of total commitment, "mak[ing] a detailed plan" (organized in terms of priority and sequence), taking immediate and specific action, and working on the plan "every single day" (note the focus on process, rather than outcomes). The last step is "resolv[ing] in advance that you will never quit," which, he states, gives you a "psychological edge." He says, "Your willingness and ability to persist are what will eventually guarantee your success."[20]

These steps, and the principles behind them, are as relevant to wellness-related goals as they are to business-related goals. They are part of the founda-tion of self-efficacy, which "correlates positively with success in all realms of personal endeavor," including patients' becoming "agents of change in their pursuit of well-being."[21] Contrary to what we may have internalized when we subjugated our own needs for sleep, self-care, and work-life balance in the interest of meeting the requirements of our medical, nursing, or other health care training, effective self-care makes us more resilient, more compassionate, and more effective in serving others, which takes us to the next important attribute of wellness success.

### Self-compassion

Meaningful healing for the dysregulated eater requires the development and ongoing practices of awareness and self-compassion. These skills, foundational to emotional intelligence and positive self-regulation, constitute an important part of the work of being an adult, even if you missed out on learning them in childhood. Many dysregulated eaters criticize their bodies harshly and berate themselves for their shortcomings when it comes to eating behaviors. Some think that relentless self-criticism and ongoing "I'm good/I'm bad" thinking, on which diet-think is predicated, will "keep them on track" around food. On the contrary, it does nothing to encourage success, and everything to destroy it.

Research by Dunkley et al., cited by Jennifer Taitz, Psy.D., in her book, *End Emotional Eating*, indicates that self-criticism actually causes suffering and is tied to anxiety, depression, and eating disorders.[22] Conversely, in an Adams and Leary study that she cites, self-compassion improves patients' ability to stay emotionally regulated, and cope better with adversity without abusing food.[23] Exercising self-compassion means accepting the body and the feelings that you have right now as the result of your best efforts to cope with life to date, rather than judgmentally criticizing yourself and engaging in negative, damaging self-talk over your "failure to achieve your goals." Kristin Neff, Ph.D., psychology researcher and self-compassion expert, describes self-compassion as "a powerful form of emotional intelligence," allowing you to be "*aware* of your feelings without being hijacked by them, so that you can make wise choices."[24] In fact, "you cannot live a happy, satisfying life without experiencing the full range of feelings—good, bad, or indifferent. If you shut them off, you're asking for trouble."[25]

Contrary to what many medical providers and dysregulated eaters have been conditioned to believe, mindful acceptance of and self-compassion for where you are at any given moment is not the same as giving up, and we as health care providers seem to have forgotten this—or perhaps we never knew it to begin with. Paradoxically, acceptance, defined as "a willingness to experience thoughts and feelings, even uncomfortable ones,"[26] is actually a first step toward change, because it allows us to take responsibility for where we are now and know that we can respond differently in the future. Those who succeed at consistently eating, exercising, resting, and striving in health-promoting ways do so in large part because they do not allow themselves to become derailed by self-sabotaging thoughts or small failures. When they eat more than they intended, or skip a workout, they respond with awareness, self-compassion, kindness, and positive, inspiring self-talk, rather than with self-criticism, knowing that they have both the responsibility and the power to continuously improve their performance, rather than head for the leftover lasagna. Thus, as

Taitz reminds us, "accepting emotions can help regulate emotions."[27] This is self-compassion and self-regulation at work, as in knowing when not to stop, but to keep going in the direction of our best life. In this way, as Taitz and Neff put it so well, "self-compassion, not self-condemnation, cultivates change,"[28] by "provid[ing] emotional resilience and enhance[ing] well-being."[29]

We know from Cognitive Behavioral Theory that actions are based upon beliefs and emotions. Mindful self-compassion allows us to feel our emotions without judging them or reacting to them with negative, downwardly spiraling self-talk. This allows us to keep our beliefs and thoughts rational and positive, which reduces feelings of overwhelm and despair when we fail to behave perfectly or achieve success (which, by the way, happens to us all). When we allow ourselves to experience our feelings, even negative ones, such as disappointment in ourselves for failing to meet our own expectations (very common with dieters) without judgment, we are able to process those feelings and not engage in psychologically self-degrading activities, such as punishing thoughts or reactive overeating.

There is a world of difference between acknowledging that you are disappointed or angry with yourself for mindlessly downing a bag of malted milk balls after a stressful day and feeling compassionate toward your own suffering, versus reacting to that same disappointment and anger by telling yourself that you are a loser and a failure who has no willpower and will never succeed at anything. In the first scenario, we are aware of our suffering and provide ourselves with a safe space to compassionately observe our feelings without piling on further pain through judgmental self-criticism. In the second scenario, we not only fail to manage the stress created by our circumstances but also add to it with our negative self-talk.

When we are compassionate toward ourselves, we can process negative or stressful feelings rationally, learn to manage them, move on, and try again (and again and again), using what we have learned. When practiced consistently, such a compassionate approach increases our psychological resilience, and we are able to continue to persevere in the face of setbacks without having to spend six months on a therapist's proverbial couch in order to recover. It also helps us to manage stress, both from external circumstances and from the reactive self-talk that poisons our minds.

Over time, practicing self-compassion allows us to spend less time wallowing in and reacting to our shortcomings, disappointments, and the results that we don't want, thus liberating mental space for us to appreciate the body that we have now and focus on what we do want. We are able to recover from negative experiences and emotions rapidly, rather than using them as an excuse to say harsh, disempowering things to ourselves—or eat mindlessly.[30] With practice, we can reclaim the mental energy that we used to spend berating ourselves and, instead, use it wisely to focus on the stepwise process of realizing our dreams. People who have a healthy relationship with their bodies and with food treat themselves with kindness, respect, and compassion. They don't demand or expect perfection of themselves 100 percent of the time, and they react to imperfection as par for the course and move on.

The result is that when these folks hit the potato chips after work, they do not talk themselves into a denigrating downward spiral that launches them into a full-fledged binge. They either eat a satisfying amount of chips guilt free or, if they overeat, give themselves retroactive permission and move on. By practicing self-compassion and the awareness that accompanies it, these successful people are often able to stop a reactive food escapade (a.k.a. binge) more quickly, which brings us to the topic of attunement. For more information on self-compassion in general and on managing emotions for dysregulated eaters, including exercises that can help patients practice this and related skills, we refer you to Kristin Neff's *Self-Compassion* and Jennifer Taitz's *End Emotional Eating*, respectively, both listed in the resources section at the end of this book.

### Attunement (to appetites as well as strengths)

Another attribute that separates those who are successful at permanently mending their relationship with food from those who live on the diet-binge seesaw is their level of attunement to their internal environment. Most high achievers, approval seekers, and people pleasers are overly attuned to the expectations and demands of the outside world, be it to the requirements of their boss or their colleagues, their spouse, parents, or children. Successful self-regulators tune in to their physical and emotional sensations, and identify them and recognize them for what they are. "Oh, that feeling in my body is fatigue. I think I'll take a short nap or rest my eyes for a minute," they'll say, rather than "I feel uneasy and overwhelmed. I need to get my work done, and I don't have time to really identify what that sensation is. I might be hungry. I'll try eating something to see if that helps, and hopefully it'll give me the energy I need to keep going with this project."

Successful self-regulators also tune into their internal hunger and satiety signals, and allow those signals to guide them in determining what, when, and how much to eat. These natural, innate (for the majority of us) cues, which many of us learned to override early on and have overridden for many years, can be reclaimed in the process of reregulating our eating habits through appetite attunement. We can also reclaim this attunement by practicing *mindful eating*, which involves cultivating nonjudgmental awareness and attending to thoughts, feelings, bodily sensations, appetite cues, and responses to food selection and eating.[31] For more information on mindfulness as it relates to eating, as well as training resources for providers, we refer you to The Center for Mindful Eating (TCME) and its website at http://www.thecenterformindfuleating.org.

And speaking of attunement, one of the most noteworthy achievements of the past several decades when it comes to promoting healthful eating practices has been the development of an evidence-based approach to appetite attunement and wellness-promoting eating behaviors, known as *Intuitive Eating*. Developed by Evelyn Tribole, M.S., R.D., and Elyse Resch, M.S., R.D., F.A.D.A., C.E.D.R.D., both experienced in the treatment of patients with eating disorders, Intuitive Eating is a lifestyle approach that promotes appetite attunement and satisfaction for the eater. A person who eats intuitively makes decisions about what and how much to eat from an internal locus of control, rather than according to an externally prescribed dietary regimen. The patient gives herself "unconditional permission to eat" in a mindful, deliberate, attuned way that promotes satisfaction, self-trust, coping with feelings without using food, and enhanced self-efficacy.[32]

The evidence for Intuitive Eating in normalizing patients' relationships with food, and promoting self-efficacy and improved health and wellness, is mounting. A recent literature review indicated that "intuitive eating is negatively associated with BMI, positively associated with various psychological health indicators, and possibly positively associated with improved dietary intake and/or healthy eating behaviours."[33] For more information, a directory of Certified Intuitive Eating Counselors, and additional training and certification opportunities for providers wishing to utilize intuitive eating principles to help their patients by becoming a Certified Intuitive Eating Counselor, we refer you to both the book *Intuitive Eating*, now in its third edition, and the website, https://www.intuitiveeating.com.

Learning to eat intuitively is empowering for patients because it is proof that they can trust themselves and take care of their needs by listening to and honoring internal body signals. This type of attunement and self-regulation has immense and far-reaching repercussions for other areas of well-being as well, because once attunement is achieved and self-care is a priority, the patient is then able to act in her own self-interest with greater self-efficacy in all of life. Learning (or, rather, relearning) intuitive eating is about proclaiming, "I can take care of myself!," a profound statement for people who have agonized for years with what they perceived as an impossibility.

It is important to note that successful self-regulators also are attuned to their strengths and desires. Rather than focusing on their shortcomings or what they have failed to achieve, they deliberately zero in on what they did well or what they plan to achieve. They use their innate talents and attributes to their advantage when taking on a new challenge or in reflecting upon past failures and considering how to proceed more constructively. This strength-focused approach, also known as *Appreciative Inquiry*,[34] is a foundational element of coaching psychology and success psychology, which we will discuss in more detail in Chapter 8.

### Visualization

One helpful key to success is the creative process of visualization, which has been highlighted in the success psychology literature as foundational to goal attainment for years.[35, 36] Visualization is the fun part of goal setting, and it is a useful tool for enhancing clarity and goal achievement. Just as it is difficult to attain what you have never clearly imagined, imagining a goal—be it an A on your science test or a fit body—can set the subconscious stage for realizing it. Successful people visualize not only the outcome goal (the fit, comfortable body, the exemplary lab values, the clean bill of health from the doctor) but also the individual steps required to achieve it. And in this way, these successful people are also process oriented. They visualize themselves planning, preparing and consuming a gorgeous, fresh, green salad, they imagine themselves running on the treadmill or racing around outdoors with their children or grandchildren on a bright, clear, sunny day. They envision and clarify every detail of their potential success until it resonates with and becomes part of them.[37] The process of *dreaming, designing, and clarifying* goals is another component of *Appreciative Inquiry*, to be discussed further in Chapter 8.

### Process orientation

Process orientation, another trait of successful people, has several advantages over the traditional medical advice model of focusing on problem solving toward outcomes only (the body perfect, number on the scale, or lab values). Motivational theory tells us that, in general, people are more interested in their quality of life and what they value than they are in lab numbers, for example. As Rollnick, Miller, and Butler remind us in their book, *Motivational Interviewing in Health Care: Helping Patients Change Behavior*, "it is the patient's own reasons for change, and not yours, that are most likely to trigger behavior change . . . the answers most likely lie within the patient, and finding them requires some listening."[38] It is often much more compelling for a sedentary Prince Charming, who wants to begin an exercise regimen, to consider visualizing the lifestyle choices that will enable him to climb the stairs to his ravishing Rapunzel without becoming winded than to consider what his doctor will say about his blood pressure numbers improving. Process orientation allows people to experience and prioritize the individual small steps that eventually lead to successful outcomes. In brief, people are motivated by what is important to them, and eliciting this by asking about patients' Desires, Ability, Reasons, and Need for behavior change (the "DARN" statements of Motivational Interviewing),[39] using open-ended "how" or "what" questions, can help patients progress to greater readiness for change.[40]

If they are able to remain mindful, attuned, and perhaps even enjoy the process or experience of becoming more active, for example, patients are more likely to soldier on than if activity is all about getting their BMI under 30 or lowering their LDL. Process orientation also allows patients to refine the vision and prepare for obstacles, including unconscious internal conflicts, which can then be addressed and resolved before they potentially derail the new behavior. Additionally, process orientation solidifies motivation, since visualizing the process (which is usually a synonym for work, commitment, or temporary discomfort, and not just arriving at the big, beautiful goal) requires a person to consider why they want this particular goal so badly and so quickly.[41]

### Positive expectations

Well-being actually may be a more important determinant of wellness success than perfect lab values or an ideal weight on the scale, because well-being encompasses the moods, motivation, and positive outlook that fuel persistence and resiliency. It is consistent, sustained behavior that determines our outcomes. Resiliency, our positive expectation that repeated commitment to values-driven processes and goals will yield benefits, and willingness to persist in the face of adversity may be the fundamental attributes that separate those who succeed and thrive from everyone else.

In his book, *Psychology of Success*, Dr. Dennis Waitley reminds us that "success is a journey, not a destination. . . . You engage in living successfully on a daily basis."[42] The same could be said of well-being. He imparts to us that "life-long success has several important ingredients . . . positive habits of thought and action that . . . [include] self-awareness . . . self-direction, self-esteem, self-discipline, self-motivation . . . and positive thinking and relationships."[43] In order for eating behaviors, which are important drivers of well-being and weight over the long term, to normalize or improve permanently, there must be an *ongoing practice* of mindfulness (defined as the "non-judgmental awareness of what is happening in the present moment"),[44] deliberate, self-directed, positive habits and self-talk, and a shift inside the mind of the patient to an internal locus of control that generate the behaviors that determine these outcomes. As discussed previously, people are much less concerned with numbers than they are with their personal values, and *only when wellness becomes a core value* will the patient assume the responsibility to set clear, effective goals and act in his or her own best interest without prodding and cajoling from a doctor, diabetes educator, dietitian, or anyone else.

### Persistence

Persistence is a measure of sustained behavior. It is defined as "the firm or obstinate continuance in a course of action in spite of difficulty or opposition."[45] It is a trait that can be either destructive or constructive. When we keep driving in a blinding blizzard in spite of the fact that we can't see the car in front of us just because "we want to get there," we're not using our best judgment. We'd be better off pulling off the road until it gets plowed or the snow lightens up. The same is true if we're running a marathon and start to experience pain in our chest. Sure, we'd love to finish the race, but we also want to live long enough to compete again if we're smart. Pushing and overdoing to get something done are examples of persistence gone awry.

However, persistence can be our friend when we apply it to improving behavior and staying self-regulated. We do this by being dogged, reminding ourselves often that we have a worthwhile goal, appreciating how far we've come, telling ourselves how great we'll feel when we have accomplished our task, visualizing whatever we're doing as successfully completed, and being our own best cheerleaders. Persistence is, more than anything, rooted in ongoing, positive self-talk and effective planning and pacing (part of the all-important skill of self-regulation).

It may have a hint of "I'll show 'em" and not wanting to disappoint others. This is fine as long as we're not all about approval seeking and proving our worthiness to ourselves or others. The best reason to persist is because confidence and self-efficacy ("the belief that one has the ability to initiate or sustain a desired behavior"[46]) grow from repeated successful action. Persisting toward a goal becomes easier when our goals are clear and aligned with our deepest values.

### Consistency

Related to persistence, one of the biggest barriers preventing dysregulated eaters from reaching their goals is a lack of consistency with their well-intentioned efforts to change their behaviors in a way that promotes sustainable wellness. They engage in a new behavior—take a walk at lunch time, relax for 10 minutes when they arrive home from work, make sure to eat breakfast, or write a shopping list before they head for the market—sometimes but not all the time. They might do it for a week or a month and stop, or they might change their behavior from one day to the next.

To build habits, we must engage in the behavior we wish to have *all the time*. That tells our brain this is what we desire to happen, and allows the basal ganglia, a part of the brain responsible for habit formation, to turn those repeated behaviors into habit.[47, 48] Difficult as learning new behavior can be, we want to make sure not to confuse our poor brains by doing *this*, then turning around and doing *that*. It is repetition, context, and consistency over time (usually longer than patients—or doctors—expect or would like) that allow new learned behaviors to become habits, solidifying new, neural pathways and allowing old ingrained habits to atrophy and fade.[49] If we only engage in a new behavior, say, sitting down while learning to eat mindfully, occasionally, we will be reinforcing both this behavior and also reinforcing old, unhealthy habits, such as eating while working on the computer, watching TV, or checking our phone messages. This dynamic is commonly known as a stand-off, and no progress will be made unless the new behavior is practiced consistently (far more often than the old one), and the change is implemented consistently for a certain period of time. In short, change only happens when we practice the new behavior more often (lots more often) than the old behavior.

Another barrier to consistency is that ongoing focused effort can wear us out. Patients will come in and tell you that they *have* been going to the gym and can't figure out why they are not seeing progress. What they're not telling you is that they have been going, but not consistently: that one week they go three times, another they go once for a half hour, and yet another week, they don't go at all. They see themselves as being compliant with what is going to lead them to good health, while you see them as not doing enough or not doing it consistently.

Please do not panic. It is not your job to teach patients how to be consistent or self-regulatory. You have enough on your plate. For now, it is sufficient for you to understand the skills they often lack when trying to become more regulated, mindful eaters and consummate caretakers of their bodies. This understanding in itself will help you be more empathic and compassionate toward them. Hopefully, it will also help you be more compassionate toward yourself and the enormous challenge you've been up against.

In Chapter 8, we will do two things. First we will detail how to use proven psychological strategies and techniques to support your patients with eating problems, guiding them toward greater mental and physical wellness. Second, we will provide you with existing and emerging resources to support these efforts without adding more hours to your day.

---

Brain food for providers: Do your patients who struggle with eating and weight concerns have many of these competencies for success? Which do most of them lack? How could you help them recognize their importance and reinforce them in your office appointments?

---

Brain food for patients: Have you ever learned about the competencies for success? Which ones do you have already, and which do you need to learn? How might you enlist your providers' help in building these competencies? How else will you learn them?

Providers, try . . .

1. Reading over the competencies for success and recognize that you and your patients both need them if you are to help your patients who have eating and weight concerns succeed.
2. Thinking about your patients of high weights and identifying which qualities and skills they generally appear to lack in success psychology terms.
3. Considering your own personality and character traits, which ones have helped you succeed and which ones you might benefit from cultivating in the future.
4. Not to feel pressured that it's your responsibility to teach life skills to your patients who suffer with body dissatisfaction, weight struggles, or eating problems.
5. Considering how hard or easy it will be for you to switch from thinking about measuring success in terms of outcomes to measuring it based upon indicators of patient well-being, including those related to awareness, self-acceptance, self-compassion, an internal locus of control, and the ability to self-regulate and respond constructively to challenges.
6. Taking time to think about how you will explain "wellness" measures and "success strategies" to your patients and how they might receive this information.
7. Talking with patients about their values and wellness vision and what kinds of support might help them connect to their goals.

Patients, try . . .

1. Determining which of your values will help you succeed at resolving your eating and weight concerns and identifying exactly why you wish to succeed in this area right now.
2. Rereading the success competencies section and considering whether there are new skills that will help you learn how to succeed.
3. Considering what your focus has been regarding wellness or weight and how that has affected your ability to succeed in attaining and maintaining your health goals.
4. Not feeling ashamed that you might not yet have mastered one or more of the skills you need and desire for success and, instead, being determined and persistent about acquiring them through practice, consistency and patience.

5. If you find that you lack many qualities for success, seriously considering working with a therapist or coach to help you develop them.
6. Shifting your focus from numbers (weight, BMI, etc.) equaling success to thinking, instead, about feeling good in your body and being proud of taking excellent care of it.

# 8

# Supporting Patients and Providers in Attaining and Maintaining Success

## (Finally, the Right Prescription!)

- Appropriate and attainable goals/outcomes for patients with eating and weight concerns
- The "weight-inclusive" approach, expressing empathy, encouraging compassion, motivational interviewing, individualizing care and goals based upon the patient's stages of change, values identification, "S.M.A.R.T." goal setting
- Additional support and training for a wellness-focused, interdisciplinary approach: Intuitive Eating community, Lifestyle Medicine, Health and Wellness Coaching
- Strategic opportunities for creative programming: culinary medicine, group work, mobilizing technology, and creating a culture of wellness in the office
- How an interdisciplinary, collaborative team approach to patient care enhances prognosis for successful, sustainable behavior change

Now that we have redefined patient success in psychological terms related to self-care, self-compassion, self-understanding, self-regulation, and life skills, you are probably wondering how to help your patients improve their skill sets, relationship with food, and their body image during a 10-minute office visit. At first glance, utilizing a psychologically based approach may seem far more complicated and burdensome than simply putting patients on a diet or prescribing an exercise regimen. However, if we are to be successful in helping patients gain competency in managing eating and weight concerns for the long term, we must empower them with strategies that are both physically and psychologically sound.

The good news is that it's not as complicated or time-consuming (or expensive) as you might expect, and you don't have to do it all yourself in a vacuum. A slew of dedicated researchers and clinicians have generated effective tools and methods that you can apply without reinventing the wheel. Please note that not all of these tools, methods, and strategies have an evidence base for this application. Where an evidence base exists or is emerging, we have noted it. We expect this to be a field of ongoing research over the next several decades, and we encourage you to track best practices and the evolution of the evidence as you implement your own approach to caring for patients with eating and weight concerns.

## IF NOT WEIGHT LOSS, WHAT ARE EFFECTIVE GOALS FOR MY PATIENTS WHO HAVE EATING AND WEIGHT CONCERNS?

As health care providers, we seek health and wellness for all of our patients, including those who struggle with eating and related health challenges. Here are seven goals that both patients and providers can pursue:

1. Optimal wellness for all of our patients, including those who struggle with overeating, body dissatisfaction, and related health challenges.
2. Consistent and sustainable implementation of wellness-promoting lifestyle behaviors, including those related to eating and nutrition, activity, sleep, stress management, life skills, and effective self-care.
3. The development of a solid psychological foundation so that patients can (with provider support) create and execute their own wellness strategy, regardless of their weight.
4. An end to the suffering, weight cycling, and associated metabolic harm[1, 2] promoted by dieting, and the development of skills to reconnect to appetite via an attuned, mindful approach such as Intuitive Eating.
5. Increased patient self-compassion for his or her current size, health, and past suffering to facilitate a greater sense of well-being and enhanced emotional resilience.[3]
6. Improved body image and acceptance of size diversity.

7. Increased self-efficacy and pride through the development of effective life and self-care skills (especially emotional regulation and stress management) and the resolution of internal psychological conflicts which may undermine lasting success.

### DO I NEED TO SPEND ANOTHER DECADE IN SCHOOL TO LEARN HOW TO HELP MY PATIENTS REACH THESE GOALS?

In a word, no. The competencies and strategies involved in creating a winning provider-patient relationship with dysregulated eaters are not at all complicated, esoteric, or even technical. In fact, we doubt they'll surprise you. Many of them are likely relational skills that you use already, albeit refined and implemented in a slightly different way, in order to enhance patients' growth, development, and success by improving their self-efficacy over time. Used flexibly and *individualized for each patient*, they comprise an integrative approach.

The following are seven skills that you can learn and develop in order to improve your relationship with and the prognosis of success for your patients with eating and weight concerns.

### First, do no harm by adopting a "weight-inclusive,"[4] wellness-focused approach, then support the development of empowering self-awareness and positive body image

When it comes to helping patients resolve dysregulated eating, we must start with the tenet to *do no harm*, particularly with children. As physicians, we naturally feel responsible for preventing and relieving suffering. In our thin-obsessed culture, nothing is guaranteed to cause needless suffering like "being too fat." Children are perceptive, and when clinicians (or parents) express concern about the number on the BMI chart, or look disappointed or annoyed when a child's weight rises "too fast," he or she often internalizes our disappointment as shame. Kids generally want to please their doctors and their parents, and when they are led to believe (through our well-intentioned alarm) that they are defective, not measuring up, or that there is something wrong with them, there can be significant, lasting psychic damage.[5]

So please give special attention to how you approach this sensitive topic with children, and feel free to refer to Tribole and Resch's *Intuitive Eating* 3rd ed.,[6] for specific approaches and evidence-based strategies to guide you. Understandably, physicians may panic because we are told that preschoolers who are at the high end of the weight continuum are five times more likely than normal-weight children to be overweight or obese as adults.[7] The truth is that healthy bodies come in a variety of shapes and sizes. Additionally, many of these children will grow taller prior to and during puberty, and with some attention to and training in self-care, attunement to appetite, and life skill development, they will be capable of remarkable psychological growth and maturity that will help them attain healthy eating habits, provided we don't destroy their self-trust and innate attunement to their internal signals first.

If we override their innate attunement to appetite cues by expressing our concern or dissatisfaction with their developing bodies, or by putting them on a restrictive diet and exercise regimen, we do two things. First, we may effectively traumatize them through the perceived deprivation that accompanies calorie restriction, which drives "seeking and overeating of restricted foods,"[8] while we also deprive them of their innate ability to tune into and trust their internal hunger and satiety signals. Second, our well-intentioned advice may promote body dissatisfaction and set up the highly motivated or approval-seeking child for overdoing exercise and seeking perfectionism in the fitness arena, thereby setting the stage for injury cycles that prevent him or her from sustaining a healthy, sane activity schedule.

We know that dieting, body dissatisfaction, and unhealthful weight control practices are a set up for weight gain and eating disorders in teens,[9] not to mention a risk factor for chronic yo-yo dieting and weight cycling in adulthood.[10] We compound the problem several-fold when we react in fear and fail to modulate our own response to that fear and concern. Leading with empathy and sensitive age-appropriate, child-centered discussion can mean the difference between despair and self-efficacy for the young patient, and hence the difference between improved health and fitness over time and a life of yo-yo dieting, disordered eating, ever-increasing weight gain, metabolic and hormonal derangement, struggle, shame, frustration, and lowered self-esteem.

With both children and adults, the first step in managing dysregulated eating and weight struggles, particularly for those who are uncomfortable with their weight, is to provide empathic, nonjudgmental listening and a sensitive initial discussion that encourages them to acknowledge and feel compassion for their own suffering, internalized weight stigma, and body dissatisfaction. Such a discussion reflects a "weight-inclusive" approach, as defined by Tylka et al. in their 2014 review article, "The Weight-Inclusive versus Weight-Normative

Approach to Health: Evaluating the Evidence for Prioritizing Well-Being Over Weight Loss."[11] Tenets of the weight-inclusive approach, which assumes that patients are "capable of achieving health and well-being independent of weight, given access to non-stigmatizing health care,"[12] include avoiding harm; appreciating size diversity; maintaining a holistic, process focus toward wellness promotion, rather than the attainment of a certain weight or BMI; incorporating sustainable, empirically supported practices into prevention and treatment efforts; emphasizing access to health-promoting foods, environments, and practices for all persons; and promoting patient autonomy and social justice.[13] Implementing a weight-inclusive approach is a way to facilitate success for our patients, rather than increasing their struggle by focusing narrowly on weight-based goals.

Before discussing weight or BMI in the presence of children, it is useful to get a sense of their body image. Inquire of children and adolescents what they appreciate most about their growing bodies and what concerns and expectations they have in the eating and weight arenas. The information gained in such an inquiry may prove useful because emerging evidence suggests that "positive body image is likely to be protective of physical health and psychological well-being" and is "positively related to intuitive eating" and other self-care behaviors.[14] Conversely, according to research cited by Bacon and Aphramor, "body dissatisfaction is associated with binge eating and other eating disordered behaviors, lower levels of physical activity and increased weight gain over time."[15] Tracy Tylka, Ph.D., and Nichole Wood-Barcalow, Ph.D., have created a ten-item comprehensive assessment of body appreciation, called the Body Appreciation Scale-2, that can be used to evaluate body appreciation and predict psychological well-being related to body image.[16] Links to this scale and other helpful evaluative tools may be found on the provider page of Dr. O'Mahoney's website at http://www.deliberatelifewellness.com.

Additionally, consider a discussion of cultural bias and unrealistic expectations concerning body size as part of preventive guidance with the eight-to-twelve-year-old set. They are sure to have opinions or questions if queried. This will help you recognize if your patient is in danger of using food and manipulation of his or her eating to resist pubertal change, able to cope with the emotional roller coaster that often characterizes adolescence, or simply considering dieting to try to fit the cultural ideal of thin. Rather than emphasizing weight or BMI, it is helpful to discuss how healthy growth promotes optimal body and brain function, encouraging a holistic approach to wellness. Implementing a "weight-inclusive" approach, as described by Tylka et al.,[17] and embodied in the Health at Every Size movement,[18] shifts the focus from weight to well-being by focusing on health promotion, lifestyle improvement, and excellent self-care for patients of any size and any age. For more information on opportunities to translate the principles embodied in a weight-inclusive approach into actual practice, we refer you to the above-referenced article by Tylka et al., and Table 1 therein, titled "Translating weight-inclusive principles into weight-inclusive practice."[19]

Taking a weight-inclusive approach with children encourages them to develop wellness-enhancing perspectives and skills early in life, which can improve their ability to care for themselves well as they navigate the transition to adulthood. And, of course, a weight-inclusive approach is an effective strategy to promote awareness, healing, and recovery for adults as well.

In terms of nutritional life skills, providers can focus discussions on how to choose the kinds of foods that fuel a strong, vibrant body and mind, and on how specific foods affect a particular patient. Age-appropriate topics might include how to identify (and prepare/pack food for older kids) whole, nutrient-dense versus nutrient-depleted, processed foods. Children can be encouraged to keep a list of breakfast foods that make them feel satisfied and support sustained energy and concentration at school, and also a list of those snack foods that result in sustained energy after an hour or two, for example. Providers can also promote attunement to internal signals[20] and emotional regulation by conversing with children about how they experience and identify internal signals of hunger and fullness, fatigue, and stress, and specific emotions (sadness, loneliness, shame, anger, anxiety, relief, joy, etc.), all of which can impact eating and coping behaviors. This is an important skill set that can support Intuitive Eating, which is associated with "both lower BMI and better psychological health."[21] The *Intuitive Eating Scale-2* "measures individuals' tendency to follow their physical hunger and satiety cues when determining when, what, and how much to eat."[22] A link to this scale may also be found on the provider page of Dr. O'Mahoney's website at http://www.deliberatelifewellness.com.

Encouraging children and adults to learn to distinguish emotional states from internal signals that indicate physical-mental needs (for fuel, water, rest, activity, relaxation, etc.) is an important step in empowering them to care for themselves, and it can help them learn how to refuel without using food when that is not what they are needing. The goal is to support emotional and body attunement and help patients develop and maintain an *internal locus of control* when it comes to their own wellness at an early age, so that they can learn to trust their ability to make choices that serve their health.

The need to first do no harm, then guide the acquisition of self-awareness is just as relevant to the preventive care of adult patients as it is to children and adolescents. Adults may not possess these skills or even recognize their importance, and you can help them tremendously by exposing them to the concepts of awareness, self-compassion, emotional regulation, internal locus of control, and self-trust. It sets the stage for patient empowerment and enhanced patient self-efficacy that can prevent dysregulated eating before it starts or mitigate it if it has already begun.

---

Brain food for providers: When you speak to patients about nutrition, do you tell them what foods are beneficial and why (as opposed to telling them only what to avoid), and do you focus on how specific foods make their bodies and minds feel? Do you generally assess patients' emotional intelligence and attunement to emotional and appetite signals as a measure of their ability to consistently and sustainably make healthy lifestyle choices?

---

Brain food for patients: What do health care providers say that supports your efforts to eat more "normally" and nutritiously? What do they say that doesn't connect, resonate with you, or that doesn't feel helpful?

---

**Harness the power of empathy with the skillful use of perceptive reflections**

By now it should come as no surprise that your patients with dysregulated eating or higher weights are actually the ones most likely to be dissatisfied with and self-critical of their body habitus and ashamed of their size. Rather than being unmotivated or complacent, most of them desperately want to improve their body image, feel better, and enjoy a satisfactory level of physical fitness and function. After repeated failures to keep weight off with restrictive dieting, however, they have suffered tremendously, not just physiologically but psychologically as well. Consequently, many of them become depressed, resentful, hopeless, and demoralized. In this state of mind, they then give up and too often turn to food to soothe their broken spirits.

Patients with this mindset can benefit enormously (far more than you would likely imagine) from empathic providers. Empathy is defined in the Wellcoaches® *Coaching Psychology Manual* as "the respectful understanding of another person's experience, including his or her feelings, needs, and desires."[23] We can feel and express empathy without necessarily sharing the same experiences, emotions, or opinions of the patient. Empathy from providers can strengthen the patient-provider relationship and encourage patients to harness and sustain internal motivation in a way that judgment, criticism, or fearmongering cannot. To quote Rollnick, Miller, and Butler, authors of *Motivational Interviewing in Health Care*, "There is very little evidence for the belief that people will change if you can just make them feel bad (scared, ashamed, humiliated) enough. To the contrary, it is the supportive, compassionate, empathic practitioner who is most effective in inspiring behavior change."[24]

So, how do you express empathy with and encourage curiosity and non-judgment in a patient who is tempted to give up on her exercise or eating plan after experiencing repeated failures in the wellness arena? By using a time-tested psychological approach pioneered by humanistic psychologist Carl Rogers, Ph.D., called *reflective listening*, or *active listening*.[25] By tuning in to how patients feel, we can then express understanding of their feelings. Expressing empathy for patients communicates acceptance and creates a safe psychological space for them to explore their beliefs and feelings about change, as well as how their "self-sabotaging" behaviors might indicate unmet needs and desires.[26]

The expression of empathy (through *reflective listening statements* or *empathy reflections*) is a powerful, learnable relational skill, rooted in Marshall Rosenberg's Nonviolent Communication (NVC) model,[27] that builds trust and, ultimately, promotes self-efficacy for the patient. As explained in the *Coaching Psychology Manual*, perceptive reflections "enable clients to hear what they are saying from the vantage point of another person . . . when coaches perceptively paraphrase and reflect what they think clients are saying, clients react with a deeper, more emotional response,"[28] which supports introspection and self-determination.

So, for example, with a patient who is considering giving up her exercise regimen due to a pattern of repeated injury, a provider could start with the statement, "I hear that you know that exercise is good for you, but that you are tired of being injured." With a patient who is mindlessly overeating to cope with being overwhelmed, you might say, "You are trying to take care of yourself with food, because everything in your life is feeling like work, you are feeling depleted, and you want to take a break and relax." With a patient who is constantly "self-sabotaging" by choosing the fast-food drive-thru over the home-prepared, nutritious meal she had planned, you might offer, "You want to eat healthfully, but after work, you feel too tired to prepare a meal." Notice that these statements are an attempt by the provider to understand and reflect how the patient is feeling without making a judgment or recommendation on how to fix the problem. This creates psychological space for patients to consider their true feelings about their situation and explore the underlying reasons for the choices they make.

Without the distraction of judgment or self-criticism, patients will then be more apt to identify (and possibly resolve) unconscious, internal conflicts about a given lifestyle choice and make a more deliberate choice about how to proceed. Thus a nonjudgmental, empathic approach encourages patient autonomy and encourages the process of change.[29] For more information on these and other powerful relational tools that enhance patients' internal motivation to change, as well as a discussion of foundational theories and methods, we refer you to the *Coaching Psychology Manual*, 2nd edition.

### Encourage patients to accept and have compassion for themselves as a tool to promote change

Compassion, as defined by Kristin Neff, Ph.D., in her book *Self-Compassion: The Proven Power of Being Kind to Yourself*, "involves the recognition and clear seeing of suffering. It also involves feelings of kindness for people who are suffering, so that the desire to help—*to ameliorate suffering*—emerges."[30] Neff explains that compassion implies absence of judgment or disdain for a person who suffers, even due to his or her own mistakes or shortcomings. According to Jennifer Taitz, Psy.D., author of *End Emotional Eating*, "self-compassion, not self-condemnation, cultivates change. . . . Self-compassion nourishes you, protecting you against emotional distress and promoting your health."[31] Thus, expressing compassion (and encouraging self-compassion) for a patient who suffers from food and eating issues is not just the right thing to do. It actually increases patients' chances of success in making lasting changes in the service of their own wellness.

You may worry that de-emphasizing weight loss and encouraging patients to be compassionate with and accepting of themselves will lead them to be complacent, self-indulgent, and lower their standards for their own behavior. Such is not the case. Taitz cites an Adams and Leary study from 2007 that demonstrated that, rather than being used as an excuse to overindulge, self-compassion led to reduced distress and decreased reactive overeating in response to "breaking their diet." "Compassion reduced distress and led to improved eating."[32]

Research cited by Kristin Neff, Ph.D., in her book *Self-Compassion*, demonstrates that "far from being a form of self-indulgence, self-compassion and real achievement go hand in hand,"[33] because self-compassion "provides the emotional safety needed to take responsibility for our actions"[34] and value ourselves enough to make "choices that lead to well-being in the long-term."[35] Self-compassion ultimately promotes self-efficacy beliefs, which enhance self-regulation and consistency in wellness-promoting behaviors. Self-criticism (and the fear and despair that it generates), on the other hand, undermines self-efficacy.[36]

Self-compassion is beneficial for both patient and provider, and is actually a first step toward developing and sustaining wellness. It helps patients become more resilient in the face of lapses or failures (such as straying from their nutritional behavioral goals) and gives them the courage to continue to strive toward their health and fitness goals, rather than self-sabotaging or giving up. Encouraging patients to practice self-compassion as part of a weight-inclusive approach[37] can be contagious, and in clinicians, maintaining compassion for patients and practicing mindful self-compassion may help to prevent burnout, promote provider wellness, and reduce stress.[38, 39] Importantly, according to Tylka et al., "empirical evidence suggests that self-compassion is an adaptive mindset to cultivate in the context of improving body image and eating behavior."[40] Moreover, how can we not feel better about ourselves when we are kind to our patients rather than when we are frustrated, aloof, critical, and shaming?

---

Brain food for providers: How do you feel about yourself when you judge patients for their failures or for not trying harder? How do you feel when you are empathic and compassionate toward them? How do they react to your attitude?

Brain food for patients: How do you feel about providers who lack compassion and invalidate your feelings and experiences? How does this affect your motivation to improve your self-care? How does provider compassion and empathy affect your motivation to become healthier?

Practicing empathy and encouraging self-compassion empowers patients to reduce their shame and quiet their negative self-talk long enough to focus on the thoughts and behaviors that lead to enhanced self-regulation, self-efficacy, and lasting change. Rather than undermining success, empathy and compassion actually facilitate success by encouraging patients to keep trying, despite circumstantial obstacles, and despite their own imperfect adherence to healthful eating and exercise, for example. It is this resilience that promotes the persistence that leads to lasting change.

We would not consider this discussion of empathy and compassion to be complete if we did not mention the importance of providers engaging in self-compassion and self-reflection. Applying these principles to our own struggles and shortcomings actually makes us more resilient and relatable. By knowing ourselves, we increase our effectiveness by relating to patients in a more humane and compassionate manner.

### Practice motivational interviewing and active listening methods and techniques

One effective way to start the conversation with patients, regardless of where they are on the readiness-for-change spectrum is through the skillful use of motivational inquiry (MI) and appreciative inquiry (AI) techniques. MI is an evidence-based counseling method, developed by William R. Miller, Ph.D., and Stephen Rollnick, Ph.D., that works by "activating patients' own motivation for change and adherence to treatment."[41] Motivational Interviewing techniques, as described in the *Coaching Psychology Manual*, include expressing empathy, developing discrepancy through open-ended inquiry, dealing with resistance effectively, and supporting self-efficacy.[42] Originally utilized within the addiction field, MI has now been applied to an expanded range of health-related behaviors. Coaching psychology incorporates MI as a method for eliciting and supporting patients' autonomous motivation and self-efficacy for change, which helps support sustainable behavioral improvement.

According to Ellen Glovsky, Ph.D., R.D., L.D.N., editor *of Wellness, Not Weight: Health at Every Size and Motivational Interviewing*, "The concepts and techniques of Motivational Interviewing work beautifully with a non-diet and HAES approach. The basic approach of MI is that practitioners enhance motivation for change in health behavior by helping clients examine their own motivation for change, and then decide if, when and how they will change." Rather than being the change agent, "the practitioner is a guide who helps them make decisions about change."[43] Motivational interviewing by a skillful provider also helps the patient become aware of and verbalize ambivalence, which, as mentioned previously, is an important first step toward resolving internal conflicts that can otherwise lead to self-sabotage or inconsistency in sustaining wellness-related behaviors.

It takes time and practice to master the techniques that form the basis of MI, but the information elicited (and the improved relationship it engenders between patient and provider) can pay huge dividends in terms of patient compliance, and can actually save time in the long run.[44] Linking goals to values is an important strategy in motivational interviewing, and wellness coaches are trained to utilize this method. Later in this chapter, we will share how wellness coaches can be powerful allies in supporting and facilitating incremental change for patients between office visits. More information on Motivational Interviewing may be found at http://www.motivationalinterviewing.org.

Appreciative Inquiry (AI) is an approach developed by David Cooperrider, Ph.D., and Diane Whitney, Ph.D.,[45] that complements motivational interviewing and is being widely applied to health care improvement efforts. AI helps patients identify their strengths and best experiences and leverage them to enhance their chances of success in reaching their goals. For example, through skillful dialogue, a practitioner might ask the patient who struggles to incorporate daily activity into his or her life when he or she has achieved success in doing it in the past. Alternatively, by asking a patient to share how he or she has overcome similar obstacles or achieved success in other contexts (work, family, community) in the past, a provider can guide a patient to identify possible strategies that he or she may not have considered applying to wellness behaviors. A patient might recall that creating a detailed plan for each week helped her to manage a large ongoing architecture project with her team at work. Applying that strategy to fitting exercise into her day can tip the balance toward success for her, by promoting her autonomy and by reminding her of her own past successes. It is also empowering, because it comes from within, rather than being forced upon her as advice. In this way, "AI encourages clients to be creative by imagining, articulating, and designing their dreams for the future . . . generating the energy for change."[46] More on how the AI approach can be applied to wellness-promoting behavioral change, including the "5-D Cycle" of transformation, can be found in the *Coaching Psychology Manual*, 2nd ed., listed in the resources section at the back of this book.

**Consider the patient's stage of change in order to individualize your treatment approach to promote patient autonomy and need recognition**

In order to help ourselves and our patients who have suffered repeated cycles of striving and failure with weight loss and weight regain, it helps to have an understanding of the transtheoretical model of change. The Transtheoretical Model of behavioral change was developed by Dr. James Prochaska and colleagues.[47] It explains that change is a process, and that helping patients identify where they are in the stages of change vastly enhances their chances of success in implementing and sustaining health-promoting behaviors. This process of stage identification also helps providers who are trained in the model identify which approaches, strategies, and types of goals will likely prove most effective for the patient or client at that particular stage.[48] The stages of change are as follows:

- Precontemplation (patients are not yet ready for change, because they are unwilling or feel that they cannot change)
- Contemplation (patients are thinking about change)
- Preparation for change
- Action
- Maintenance[49]

A working knowledge of Prochaska's Transtheoretical Model of Change can be particularly useful when caring for dysregulated eaters and chronic dieters, because people who have failed multiple times at weight loss end up subconsciously not believing that they have the ability to change (precontemplation), even though, in their conscious mind, they are "trying" (action). They may attempt to implement changes in their behavior and make wellness-promoting choices, but they "self-sabotage" or become easily frustrated or thwarted by obstacles, because, at a subconscious level, they have become disempowered and demoralized and are not yet ready to try again.

These patients need to work on identifying and processing their beliefs, feelings (including mixed feelings), and thoughts about their goals, prior to implementing behaviors.

They will also benefit greatly from working with a skilled coach or therapist who understands motivation and how to help guide them from precontemplation to contemplation, where they achieve conscious awareness of their internal conflicts and ambivalence about success. The truth is that most patients initially are motivated to improve their eating behaviors and remain remarkably motivated until they experience repeated failures through dieting and/or injuries due to overexercising. Then they often cease to believe that change is possible for them. They are effectively back in precontemplation without realizing it. They may continue the cycle of trying and failing without realizing that they lack the psychological foundation and understanding of the change process for success.

For more information on the Transtheoretical Model and the psychology of behavior change, we refer you to Wellcoaches® *Coaching Psychology Manual*, 2nd edition, and to http://www.prochange.com, both in the resources section at the end of this book.

### Encourage patients to explore and define their values and also to view past failures as opportunities for learning and personal growth

Helping patients recognize that they are stuck in precontemplation is one of the most potentially empowering things that you can do for them. Rather than focusing on behaviors, these patients benefit from doing thinking and feeling work around their behavioral goals.[50] This process has the added benefit of helping patients clarify their values and goals (a key competency from success psychology) and resolve mixed feelings.[51] Helping patients identify their core values and how these values apply to their wellness goals is another way to empower them. While you can plant the seeds of change during an office visit, cultivating a vision and a plan for wellness-promoting behavior change takes time. So does learning from past failures and frustrations by identifying the needs that must be met and the ambivalence that must be resolved for change to be sustainable for a given patient.

For this reason, referring patients to a certified lifestyle medicine or health and wellness coach, or to a dietitian, therapist, or other clinician trained in Intuitive Eating and behavioral change, can be life-changing for the patient. Many of these experts are trained to facilitate and support constructive, incremental, ongoing behavior change for patients in this situation, and they have the time to devote to that critically important process. Once patients have had an opportunity to do this work with a coach or therapist, their readiness to implement your behavioral recommendations increases immeasurably.

Information on training opportunities for clinicians and referral resources may be found later in this chapter and in the resources section at the end of this book. Additionally, you may download worksheets that you can use to encourage patient awareness and start the conversation about readiness for change from the provider page of Dr. O'Mahoney's website, http://www.deliberatelifewellness.com.

### Learn effective goal-setting techniques to help patients keep their goals S.M.A.R.T.

Health and wellness coaches are trained to help patients set goals that are *specific, measurable, action-based, realistic, and time-bound.*[52] This technique, borrowed from the business literature and attributed to George Doran,[53] encourages the creation of goals for which progress can be evaluated based upon the specific measures, as outlined above. Framing and refining goals to make them S.M.A.R.T. helps patients to be very clear and specific about their goals and also makes them mindful of the small, incremental steps, potential obstacles, and consistent and sustained action (self-regulation) that will be necessary to achieve them. Framing goals in this way (and writing them down) promotes success by encouraging ongoing evaluation of progress according to specific, measurable criteria, according to experts in success psychology.[54]

In the health professions, we tend to focus on measurable outcomes when we recommend goals to our patients, because this is what medical research often assesses and tracks. However, there are other types of goals that patients and providers can focus on to enhance their patients' chances of success with the outcome goals. These include cognitive goals, such as thinking about the pros and cons of change versus those of staying the same, identifying feelings about a potential behavioral change, including ambivalence/conflicted feelings (e.g., wanting to start an exercise regimen in order to improve health, but also not wanting to commit to it because it is time-consuming and has not resulted in a trimmer body in the past), behavioral goals, skill goals, and goals related to improving self-trust, self-confidence, self-pride, consistency, and perseverance (self-regulation). By learning how to help patients identify appropriate goals for both their stage of change and refine their goals to be S.M.A.R.T., you provide them with the ability to evaluate their progress objectively, toward goals that resonate with their values and vision for their best life. More information on S.M.A.R.T. goal setting may be found in the resources section of this book, and in the *Coaching Psychology Manual.*[55]

### Established and emerging resources for support and collaboration

Working with collaborative providers from different disciplines provides patients with resources and skills to improve their emotional intelligence (the ability to identify, express, and manage feelings effectively), which has been shown to correlate with both health and success.[56] By engaging in deliberate self-development and by learning to prioritize and engage in effective self-care, either on their own or in conjunction with therapy or coaching, patients are able to develop the life skills and resilience that support a consistent practice of wellness-promoting beliefs, thoughts, and behaviors. We recommend that you familiarize yourself and your colleagues with the following emerging resources that will help patients improve on implementing your professional recommendations, based upon their individual situation.

### The Intuitive Eating and Health at Every Size® communities

As you seek support and resources to help your patients achieve success in overcoming dysregulated eating, we encourage you to investigate the Intuitive Eating and Health at Every Size® (HAES) Communities. Providers and qualified staff may obtain targeted training in helping patients achieve eating attunement and related self-care skills through the Intuitive Eating ProSkills Intensive teleseminar. Information for both providers and patients may be accessed at https://www.intuitiveeating.com.

Pioneered by Linda Bacon, Health at Every Size® is an evidence-based, weight-inclusive approach that encourages the promotion of health (rather than weight management) respect for body diversity, and compassionate self-care. According to Bacon and Aphramor, "Randomized Controlled clinical trials indicate that a HAES approach is associated with statistically and clinically relevant improvements in physiological measures (e.g. blood pressure, blood lipids), health behaviors (e.g. eating and activity habits, dietary quality) and psychosocial outcomes (such as self-esteem and body image), and that HAES achieves these health outcomes more successfully than weight loss treatment and without the contraindications associated with a weight focus."[57] A fact sheet on the HAES approach, as well as additional information, may be found through the Association for Size Diversity and Health (ASDAH) at https://www.sizediversityandhealth.org/content.asp?id=161.

Both organizations offer support communities for patients as well as resources, education for providers, and information for others interested in the ongoing research in this area.

### Leverage the best evidence and practices from Lifestyle Medicine

As we strive to help patients improve their abilities to better care for themselves and achieve improved health outcomes, we have the opportunity to integrate an emerging source of education, support, and evidence-based best practices to help us. This is the relatively new field of Lifestyle Medicine. According to the American College of Lifestyle Medicine, "eighty percent or more of all healthcare spending in the U.S. is tied to the treatment of conditions rooted in poor lifestyle choices. Chronic diseases and conditions—such as hypertension, heart disease, stroke, type 2 diabetes, obesity, osteoporosis, multiple types of cancer—are among the most common, costly and preventable of all health conditions."[58] In an effort to address and reverse this trend, lifestyle medicine practice focuses on utilizing lifestyle interventions related to nutrition, physical activity, stress reduction, rest, smoking cessation, and avoidance of alcohol abuse as first-line therapy, for prevention, treatment, and reversal of chronic disease.[59]

Behavioral change counseling in the interest of promoting improved health and quality of life is thus an important part of this approach, and lifestyle medicine education initiatives, including the Lifestyle Medicine Education Collaborative, seek to enhance medical trainees and practitioners' competency in this area.[60] This is an exciting movement, because it makes proven behavioral change techniques and psychology-based strategies available to medical trainees and providers that they might not have had access to in the past—an empowering skill set to offer patients. More information for providers may be found at http://lifestylemedicineeducation.org/.

According to David Katz, M.D., M.P.H., president of the American College of Lifestyle Medicine, "Lifestyle as medicine has the potential to prevent up to 80% of chronic disease; no other medication can match that. It's free of all but good side effects and is safe and appropriate for children and octogenarians alike. It is, quite simply, the best medicine we've got."[61] By adding competency in lifestyle medicine and success psychology to our toolbox, or by committing to maintaining a network of high-quality referral providers with this expertise, we have the potential to help millions who have not been helped—or have even been hurt—by business-as-usual diet-and-exercise advice.

The only reference to a "dream team" you may recall is the legal squad that was pulled together during the O. J. Simpson trial in 1995. Well, medicine can have its dream team as well, in the service of health promotion. The "Dream Team" approach, as described at the June 2015 Lifestyle Medicine Conference hosted by Harvard Medical School,[62] has the potential to save time and money, and it may help prevent both patient and practitioner burnout in the long run. The "dream team" includes a physician trained in lifestyle medicine, a lifestyle medicine or health and wellness coach, a mental health provider or therapist, a dietitian, and an exercise physiologist, optimally all under one roof, for convenience and continuity of patient care. For patients who suffer from dysregulated eating behaviors, this interdisciplinary collaborative model holds exciting potential for streamlining the process of healing and improving self-care. It can provide patients with unprecedented access to providers with complementary skill sets, enabling them to make more rapid progress than they could working with you alone (no matter how caring and competent you are).

Several top medical schools are offering fellowships in lifestyle medicine for physicians seeking additional training in this new specialty, and, as mentioned previously, a Lifestyle Medicine Education Collaborative has been formed to include training in Lifestyle Medicine for medical students.[63] This is a burgeoning area of health care and wellness promotion, which we believe will be integral to successful medical practice in the future. We hope that the psychology of eating approach outlined in this book will help to advance the state of the art and become standard practice in lifestyle medicine and wellness coaching when treating dysregulated eaters. Additional information may be found through the American College of Lifestyle Medicine at http://www.lifestyle-medicine.org and at http://lifestylemedicineeducation.org.

Brain food for providers: How open are you to learning about Lifestyle Medicine? How much does it speak to your treatment needs with patients who struggle with overeating and weight concerns? How open are you to the concept of working with a "dream team"? Do you fear you don't have the time, that you don't know the kind of professionals you would include in such a team, or that you might lose control of treatment decisions?

Brain food for patients: What is your reaction to working with a team of providers who can help you with the psychological and physical aspects of resolving your eating and weight concerns? Are you thinking this might be too much of a time and energy commitment for you or that this is just what the doctor ordered?

### Health and Wellness Coaches: An emerging resource for helping patients implement and sustain health-promoting practices

The good news is that, despite the fact that you as a clinician are unlikely to have the time to do all of this work personally with your patient, the evolving discipline of coaching psychology can provide practical support for helping patients build a psychological foundation for persistence and success in reaching and sustaining their goals. Coaches can provide much-needed support for patients who do not otherwise suffer from psychological dysfunction. For patients who suffer from dysregulated eating with psychological dysfunction, a referral to an appropriate mental health professional is necessary. Maintaining a referral network of qualified providers, including certified health and wellness coaches, certified Intuitive Eating counselors, and eating disorders therapists, can provide you with appropriate, patient-specific sources of collaborative support for helping your patients improve their eating, self-care behaviors, and wellness-related outcomes.

The National Consortium for the Credentialing of Health and Wellness Coaches (NCCHWC) defines the coach as "a professional trained in evidence-based motivational strategies, behavior change theory and processes, healthy lifestyle knowledge and powerful communication techniques that assist clients (or patients) to develop inner resources and intrinsic motivation for sustaining lifestyle improvement, and health and well-being."[64] National training and education standards leading to NCCHWC certification are designed to ensure that health and wellness coaches have the specific skills to help patients in a constructive, safe, progressive manner.[65] Not surprisingly, health and wellness coaches usually have a background in the health and wellness professions. They may be registered nurses, dietitians, psychotherapists, diabetes educators, other mental health providers, athletic trainers, or even physicians, who undertake additional training in behavior change theory and coaching psychology.

Wellness coaches work to promote clients' autonomous motivation, self-efficacy, and self-regulation skills, attributes which support successful, sustained behavioral and wellness improvement. Based upon a recent systematic review, these three attributes "emerge as the most promising individual-level mediators of positive weight outcomes and increased physical activity."[66] Emerging evidence demonstrates that coaching improves client-patient outcomes, compliance, employee health, and productivity, and may lower health care costs.[67] This specialized training, in combination with a weight-inclusive approach[68] to wellness, holds tremendous promise for our patients in healing dysregulated eating.

According to Margaret Moore, M.B.A., CEO of Wellcoaches® corporation, who in 2002 founded the first coaching school for health and wellness professionals and since then has been instrumental in establishing a coaching science foundation in the United States, "certified Health and Wellness Coaches are uniquely qualified. . . . The coaching curriculum is science-based, integrating 15 evidence-based theories and domains in behavior change and coaching psychology."[69] Certified health and wellness coaches receive strategic training in behavior change and success-promoting, client-centered strategies that transcend disciplines. Most health care providers are not exposed to this approach in their medical, nursing, dietetics, or other training. If you would like to learn more about training opportunities, or to find a certified health and wellness coach in your area, you may refer to the NCCHWC at http://www.ncchwc.org/, or to the Wellcoaches® website at http://www.wellcoachesschool.com/. Additionally, Wellcoaches® has recently published the second edition of the *Coaching Psychology Manual*, which describes the theoretical foundations of coaching psychology, along with evidence-based coaching protocols.

A compelling example of how interdisciplinary collaboration can increase our ability to help our patients, Wellcoaches® and the American College of

Lifestyle Medicine recently established a partnership to "co-develop Lifestyle Medicine and Healthy Behaviors Curriculum for Health and Wellness Coaches."[70] According to David Katz, M.D., M.P.H., president of the American College of Lifestyle Medicine, "Coaches reach an enormous number of people, and, with standardized training in lifestyle medicine, they'll have an enhanced ability to promote health and prevent disease. The public can be confident that certified coaches are practicing at a high standard and providing evidence-based guidance. Certified Health and Wellness Coaches who specialize in lifestyle medicine will become integral members of the lifestyle medicine practice team, contributing importantly to the treatment and even reversal of disease." Moreover, "A national standard for health coaching in [the area of lifestyle medicine] will . . . [allow] many more people to benefit from the opportunity lifestyle medicine uniquely offers: adding years to our lives, and life to our years."[71] Additional information on health and wellness coaching and the Lifestyle Medicine/Wellcoaches® collaboration can be found at http://well-coachesschool.com and http://www.lifestylemedicine.org.

## MORE STRATEGIES FOR CLINICIANS TO HELP PATIENTS SUCCEED
### Think outside the box—and inside the "teaching kitchen"

Another option, provided that space is available, is to offer access to a "teaching kitchen" for staff and patients. This concept was introduced and the advantages beautifully explained in a 2015 article by David Eisenberg, M.D., and Jonathan Burgess,[72] and in a 2016 summary of emerging programs by Rani Polak, M.D., Chef, M.B.A., et al.[73] The idea behind teaching kitchens and culinary medicine programs is that providers are more likely to provide useful counsel to patients on nutritious eating if they themselves have been exposed to strategies for success in meal planning, procurement of ingredients, and preparation. For this reason, lifestyle medicine programs, medical schools, and hospital systems are starting to provide culinary medicine training to providers and patients.[74]

In an office-based setting, the teaching kitchen could be a break room or even the waiting room of an office after office hours, where meal planning and simple preparation classes (assembling previously cooked and frozen items into a salad, for example) could be made available to staff and patients. Such classes would not only contribute to patients' self-efficacy in the kitchen but also provide ideas and techniques for planning and assembling a high-nutrient-density meal for people who want to eat better but lack the time and skill set to plan and execute one. The physician's office is a trusted, accessible venue for many people, and making these services available to patients during or outside of office hours can serve to maximize access for the patient and revenue for the practice.

We expect that you must be wondering how you can possibly integrate these ideas into your already hectic schedule, particularly with limited time to see each patient and the lack of insurance reimbursement for counseling-based services. By integrating a collaborative interdisciplinary approach based upon lifestyle medicine principles with a group therapy–based model and a little help from twenty-first-century technology, we can help patients achieve consistency and persistence in wellness-promoting behaviors in an efficient manner. At the same time, we can control costs by providing information-based services to more than one person at a time and outside of office hours. What follows are some possible options for consideration within the constraints and resources of your individual practice situation.

### Harness the power of groups and workshops

In the 1970s, psychotherapist Susie Orbach published the groundbreaking book, *Fat Is a Feminist Issue*, in which she recommended a support group model for helping emotional eaters.[75] The group model has been proven to work through programs like Alcoholics Anonymous and in both inpatient and outpatient eating disorder treatment programs, which provide support, psychoeducation, and a new social norm to persons who are in recovery. In our current health care environment, counseling services by physicians, for example, are poorly reimbursed. Moreover, barriers to mental health services (based upon both access and cost) are significant.

In this economic context, the group model saves money in multiple ways. First, the clinician need not repeat the same information over and over. Second, the group setting allows people to process their experiences and feelings at different rates over time within a supportive context, a luxury which is rarely available in a 10-minute physician visit. Third, it facilitates access, even for those with limited economic means, by allowing each participant to pay a smaller amount out of pocket, while still allowing the provider to receive an hourly rate sufficient to keep the lights on and the office running.

Opportunities for implementing the group model to help patients build a psychoeducational foundation for success are limited only by your imagination. Practices can hire or collaborate with a therapist or coach experienced in group work to facilitate weekly sessions covering a rotating curriculum of topics of interest to those in recovery from dysregulated eating. Education and transformational discussion could thus take place outside of (or even during) office hours, allowing patients to experience growth and progress between clinician visits. Coordinating the group's curriculum with the patient's stage of change and running several weekly groups for patients at different stages could help to further differentiate the group curriculum and meet patients where they are.

For an even simpler and more cost-effective approach, you could start a book club for patients of your practice, using books that deal with dysregulated eating, body image, etc. The book club could meet at set intervals either during or outside of office hours and could be facilitated by a staff member trained in counseling, motivational interviewing, Intuitive Eating, or health and wellness coaching. Examples of cost-effective training programs and opportunities for further reading may be found in the resources section at the end of this book.

### Use technology to promote wellness

By combining tools from eating psychology and coaching psychology with twenty-first-century technology, we have the ability to combine forces with other experts and design classes and workshops for our patients that will help them implement our best advice. For practices with a wide catchment area, or for populations with transportation challenges, other strategies for patient psychoeducation during nonoffice hours exist. For example, a lifestyle medicine-trained clinician or multidisciplinary group could collaborate with a registered dietitian or culinary medicine-trained chef to create group e-mail blasts or YouTube videos on various wellness-promoting topics, and e-mail the links weekly to interested patients.

Potential topics for group e-mails or videos could include meal planning techniques to maximize nutrient density and minimize waste on a budget, suggestions for safe physical activity options that bring pleasure and where to find them in the area, and alternatives to food-seeking for comfort. Additional tools for disseminating information and providing relational support for patients include Skype/VSee group sessions, webinars or Google hangouts, or other social media resources. Validated scales from cutting-edge researchers in this area can be used to measure patient progress. Links to these and other resources may be found on the providers page of Dr. O'Mahoney's website at http://www.deliberatelifewellness.com.

### Institute some climate change in your office

Still another potentially empowering and cost-effective idea is creating an office culture that encourages both staff and patients to combine wellness-related behaviors with involvement in something larger than themselves. This is a very real way to help patients cultivate meaning and purpose by helping others while incorporating physical activity and self-care into their lives. Staff and/or patients might train with others to walk, bike, or run a 5K to raise money for ALS, cancer, MS, or diabetes research, or form a crafting group to knit blankets for babies in the NICU or make jewelry for women returning to work. Walk With a Doc is an example of community-based effort that combines community-based patient education with exercise.[76] These group-based, community-building activities serve a dual purpose. They create community around fun, altruistic physical activity and provide a support network for staff and patients, both of which have been shown to reduce stress and improve health.[77] This contributes to the creation of a culture of mutual purpose and wellness among providers, staff, and patients.

Another option for promoting a culture of wellness in your office is to provide office staff access to training in weight-inclusive practices, lifestyle medicine topics, health and wellness coaching principles, and Intuitive Eating practices. Staff trained in such skills and methods might participate in the creation of educational materials or lead book club-type discussions for patients. Web- or video-based educational materials can be used repeatedly, updated when necessary, and shared with staff and patients alike, for a relatively small financial investment. Such an investment can improve retention and minimize costs associated with training staff in a high turnover situation. Done well, this investment also improves both efficiency and morale among the members of the treatment team, because everyone is on the same page with an important mission of the practice, and everyone has the opportunity to grow in a way that can improve not only his or her professional life but also his or her personal life.

Perfection is not required. Patients benefit from seeing providers and staff walk the walk, increase their own wellness, work to overcome obstacles and, by cultivating resilience, maintain progress. In fact, accepting imperfection and seeing others strive facilitates trust and communication and cohesiveness among providers and patients, which can't help but improve care and promote change for the better.

You may not be able to help every dysregulated eater with this proposed approach, but you are likely to at least *do no harm,* and it is probable that more of your patients will be well-served by this approach than were served with restrictive diets that rarely can be sustained and which studies tell us are bound to fail for the long term. Moreover, the general trajectory of progress will finally be headed in the right direction, as patients increase their awareness, self-care and life skills and stop unconsciously sabotaging their own best efforts. After all, as the first law of holes states, "If you find yourself in a hole, stop digging."[78]

We hope that this information has been illuminating and will be empowering for both you and your patients in treating the causes and finding individualized solutions to dysregulated eating. What we offer is an innovative approach to improving patient care and outcomes through a weight-inclusive,[79] psychologically oriented paradigm. Our goal is to reduce weight and fat stigma, investigate best practices to promote patient empowerment and self-efficacy, and to provide strategies for success and support to patients and to the providers who care for them.

Doctors and health care providers can make an enormous difference in the lives of their patients with eating and weight concerns. However, a prescription for even the most optimal nutrition or exercise regimen will likely fail to improve our patients' health long-term if they lack the self-efficacy, internal locus-of-control, and persistence to implement *and sustain* the behaviors that promote lasting wellness. This is done by encouraging patients to make a cognitive shift to sustainable self-care by connecting to their emotions, appetites, and personal reasons for lifestyle improvement. By asking change-promoting questions and collaborating across disciplines, we have an opportunity to support patients' commitment to their own wellness and to taking charge of their health.

Providers, try . . .

1. Practicing being an active listener, a good empathizer, and having compassion for your patients at whatever weight, level of wellness, or stage of change they are in.

2. Focusing less on weight and other outcomes measures and more on the process of how they will get there.

3. Making sure that you are not clinging to the idea that diets work for the long term just because you think that learning and implementing new strategies may be difficult, cost-prohibitive, or time-consuming.

4. Being compassionate with yourself for not doing your job perfectly, with the expectation that learning and implementing the psychology of success strategies in this chapter will take time and will ultimately improve the quality of your patient care and your relationships with patients.

5. Imagining what kind of a "dream team" you could put together, including getting ideas from colleagues on competent professionals they have consulted.

6. Being open with your patients who have eating and weight concerns about the fact that you are changing your approach to treating them and welcome their ideas and feedback.

7. Learning more about lifestyle medicine competencies and practices on the ILM website at http://www.instituteoflifestylemedicine.org/.

Patients, try . . .

1. Learning more about lifestyle medicine and health and wellness coaching through the websites http://www.lifestylemedicine.org/ and http://www.ncchwc.org/.

2. Telling your physician or health care provider if you believe that you would benefit from more support for psychological and behavioral changes related to improving your relationship with food.

3. Thinking about why you're afraid to give up dieting and discussing your feelings with your health care provider.

4. Considering consulting a certified health and wellness coach who understands Intuitive Eating and Health at Every Size principles for coaching on eating or health goals, making an appointment with a registered dietician, hiring a qualified fitness coach, scheduling a session with an eating disorders therapist, or finding a group to support positive changes in your eating and lifestyle choices.

# Our Stories

## KAREN'S "STORY"

Before I had my tonsils removed at five or six years old in the early 1950s, my parents played the train game to woo me to eat. "Open the tunnel," they'd coax. "Here comes the train!" And when I finally opened my mouth, they'd slip the food into it, look at each other, and sigh with relief. Then, in the hospital after my tonsillectomy, I fell in love with the ice cream the nurses offered me, wanting as much of it as I could get. A few short years later, my mother was shopping for me in the chubby girls' section of the department store. Suddenly, I loved food and had become what in those days was called (and maybe still is) a "good" eater.

Here's how being a "good" eater turned into becoming a dysregulated one. My average-weight mother was a normal eater and passable cook who served my father and me balanced, healthy meals. Dad, who passionately enjoyed food and tended to yo-yo 10 pounds or so up and down the scale, was a member of the clean-plate club. He'd sit at the table reading the *New York Telegram* until I finished all the food on my plate, e-v-e-r-y l-a-s-t m-o-r-s-e-l. He insisted—no discussion!—that I try every food I was given and eat disgusting things like gristle and the strings from inside the banana peel which made me gag. My mother wouldn't allow me to open a box of food until a previous box was finished: eat the Cheerios and only *then* open the Corn Flakes, and don't open the Oreos *until* you're done with the Vanilla Wafers. You get the picture.

As a preadolescent, I remember her chastising me on more than one occasion because I ate the whole jar of maraschino cherries after she'd warned that she was saving them for "company" that night. And I recall wondering, didn't I deserve them too, and why couldn't she have bought one jar for us and one for "company"? To outsmart her, I became a sneak eater and went from a chubby child to a self-conscious, chubby teenager. During my adolescence, I alternated between near-starvation ("Hurray," I wrote in my diary, "I only ate an apple today!") and being what I call a world-class binge eater. By college, I could eat a quart of ice cream in a sitting and had contests with the girl in the dorm room next to me to see who could finish one first.

By my 20s, bingeing and overeating had become a way of life, interspersed with rigidly self-enforced caloric restriction. At five feet tall, my weight kept inching upward. In my early 30s, working at a Boston ad agency where it seemed all the women were slim, I engaged in purging for about eighteen months and became as slim as they were. Clever girl, I thought.

Not so clever, it turned out. A friend I'd told about my bulimia urged me to seek therapy. Through counseling and reading Susie Orbach's *Fat Is a Feminist Issue*, over the next half decade, I struggled toward "normal" eating. Hopeful that I could actually create a comfortable relationship with food, I devoured every book on the subject, not that there were many back then, when the (now worldwide) nondiet movement was just taking off in the early 1980s. I dutifully practiced having "forbidden" food in my apartment until I could eat just as much as I wanted of it and not polish off entire bags or boxes all at once. I still weighed myself daily but eventually ditched the scale, finally understanding that to stay tuned into my appetite, I had to focus exclusively on eating, not weight. My weight declined gradually and I began tweaking my food intake to be nutritious as well as "normal."

After receiving an M.Ed. and an M.S.W., I began specializing in treating what I call troubled eaters, mostly of the emotional, mindless, and overeating variety. Then, by combining my eating recovery experience with my clinical training, I started writing books to spread the word on how to stop dieting and enjoy a comfortable relationship with food and body. And, today, here I am, grateful for half a lifetime of being a "normal," healthy eater.

### PAIGE'S "STORY"

My baffling battle with food, body image, and the scale started before age 10. Like many young girls of my generation and those that followed, I internalized the thin ideal early. During middle school, I thought daily about how to make my body smaller, trying to limit myself to small quantities of low-fat, diet foods and reading everything I could find about how to lose weight. For several years, I succeeded in slowing my weight gain, but by early adolescence, my weight started to escalate, and my body image worsened. At the same time, I lived with a persistent, nagging feeling of deprivation.

My experience contrasted with what I saw among my family members who managed to attain and maintain a stable, comfortable weight. My father and brother were both active and fit. My mother was petite and mightily disciplined when it came to eating. I remember watching her virtuously munching her "diet-approved" dinner of dry chicken breast and broccoli with her lemon water as I poured ranch dressing over everything on my plate. My brother and I still tease her by insisting that we had chicken breasts and broccoli for dinner five days a week for ten years in a row. That is not at all true. It just felt like it.

Despite playing sports and jogging throughout middle and high school "to keep my weight down," I continued to weight cycle. I would diet, feel deprived, binge, feel ashamed, diet, feel deprived, binge, and gain more weight through my teenage years and early 20s. I felt like a failure. Uncomfortable in my body and completely out of attunement with my true hunger and satiety signals, I believed that I could not trust myself to know what or how much to eat and that I was doomed to struggle against my body forever. I also believed that I needed to be thin to be worthy of happiness, satisfaction, respect, and love; thin like the actresses on TV, the models in "fitness" magazines, and others who seemed never to struggle with their weight.

I started my first commercial diet program at age 13. For the next thirty years, I engaged in one diet after another as my weight yo-yo'd up and down. In my teens and 20s, I remember starving myself (vowing to eat only grapefruit, or only bell peppers, or only lettuce) as a reaction to the number on the scale, then bingeing on chocolate or ice cream when the inevitable headache and fatigue overwhelmed me days or even hours later. I felt shame, confusion, and despair virtually anytime I ate anything, and thought constantly about how I could "do better" with my food and eating!

In my 30s and early 40s, by which time I was sharing a house with a husband and two children, I was committed to serving healthy, home-cooked, nutritionally balanced meals, which I also overate. While raising my family, I learned to make delicious nutrient-dense dishes. But consuming them didn't mitigate my struggle, because I was still not attuned to my hunger and satiety signals and was still engaged in counterproductive self-talk, which drove me to the ice cream carton on more than one occasion. After an overeating episode, I would exercise vigorously to try to burn off the extra calories consumed. Despite exercising on and off for decades, I had never developed a consistent activity regimen as an adult, due to a pattern of intense workouts, followed by injury, followed by no workout for weeks at a time while I healed from whatever overuse injury I had wrought.

My personal and professional accomplishments, which I believed certainly should have proven more challenging than "simply controlling my weight," seemed to pale in the face of what I saw as my most shameful failing. During medical school and residency, I wondered how I could achieve top grades in my courses and positive feedback from professors, patients, and families, and still not manage to "successfully" restrict my eating or achieve a sustainable comfortable weight. Like most medical residents at that time, I ignored my own exhaustion, hunger, thirst, and even my full bladder, for hours on end during thirty-plus-hour shifts at the hospital. I worked tirelessly to provide the best possible care to my patients at all hours of the day and night, and yet this issue of willpower, as I saw it, still eluded me.

I ultimately wound up 30 pounds heavier than when I had started dieting at age 13 before I finally resolved my dysregulated eating issues and improved my appetite attunement, body image, and self-care habits. Since then, I have gradually achieved a positive, peaceful relationship with food and now consider myself to be a "normal eater." I am comfortable in my body; I enjoy exercising gently, mindfully, and consistently most days per week; my attitude toward my body is now one of enormous gratitude; and caring for it has become a source of pride, balance, and perspective, rather than of pain. This learning process involved the acquisition of certain life skills and self-care habits that were missing from my many years of formal education.

The needless suffering that I endured during thirty years of dieting and weight cycling and the remarkable progress, healing, and hope that graced my life once I stopped obsessing about weight and learned and began to practice a new skill set are the reasons that I now devote much of my professional career to helping dysregulated eaters end the war with food, their bodies, and the scale. This book represents one such effort by providing education, perspective, and support to the physicians and health care providers who care for them.

# Notes

## INTRODUCTION

1. Rebecca Puhl, J. L. Peterson, and J. Luedicke, "Motivating or Stigmatizing? Public Perceptions of Weight-Related Language Used by Health Providers" abstract, *International Journal of Obesity (Lond)* 37 (April 2013): 612–19. doi:10.1038/ijo.2012.110.

2. Samantha Ellis, Katherine Rosenblum, Alison Miller, and Karen E. Peterson, "Meaning of the Terms 'Overweight' and 'Obese' Among Low-Income Women," *Journal of Nutrition Education and Behavior* 46, no. 4 (July–August 2014): 299–303. doi:10.1016/j.jneb.2013.08.006.

3. Tracy L. Tylka, et al., "The Weight-Inclusive versus Weight-Normative Approach to Health: Evaluating the Evidence for Prioritizing Well-Being over Weight Loss," *Journal of Obesity* (2014): 1–18, article ID 983495. http://dx.doi.org/10/1155/2014/983495.

## CHAPTER 1

1. William H. Dietz, et al., "Management of Obesity: Improvement of Health-Care Training and Systems for Prevention and Care," *Lancet* 385 (2015): 2521–33. http://dx.doi.org/10.1016/, S0140-6736(14)61748-7.

2. Kimberly A. Gudzune, Wendy L. Bennett, Lisa A. Cooper, and Sara N. Bleich, "Patients Who Feel Judged about Their Weight Have Lower Trust in Their Primary Care Providers," *Patient Education and Counseling* 97, no. 1 (October 2014): 128–31. http://dx.doi.org/10.1015/j.pec.2014.06.019.

3.  William H. Dietz, et al., "Management of Obesity," 2521–33. http://dx.doi. org/10.1016/, S0140-6736(14)61748-7.

4.  Kelly M. Adams, Martin Kohlmeier, and Steven H. Zeisel, "Nutrition Education in U.S. Medical Schools: Latest Update of a National Survey," *Academic Medicine* 85, no. 9 (September 2010): 1537–42. http://dx.doi.org/10.1097/ ACM.0b013e3181eab71b.

5.  Phyllis Glanc, et al., "Challenges of Pelvic Imaging in Obese Women," *Radiographics* 32, no. 6 (2012): 1839–62. doi: 10.1148/rg.326125510.

6.  "Obesity and Anesthesia," American Society of Anesthesiologists website, accessed August 8, 2016, https://www.asahq.org/whensecondscount/patients%20 home/preparing%20for%20surgery/surgery%20risks/obesity%20and%20 anesthesia.

7.  Yvonne N. Pierpont, et al., "Obesity and Surgical Wound Healing: A Current Review," *ISRN Obesity* (2014): 1–13. http://dx.doi.org/10.1155/2014/638936.

8.  Girish P. Joshi, et al., "Society for Ambulatory Anesthesia Consensus Statement on Preoperative Selection of Adult Patients with Obstructive Sleep Apnea Scheduled for Ambulatory Surgery," *Anesthesia and Analgesia* 115, no. 5 (November 2012): 1060–68. http://dx.doi.org/10.1213/ANE.0b013e318269cfd7.

9.  Amri Ramzi, Liliana Bordeianou, Patricia Sylla, and David Berger, "Obesity, Outcomes and Quality of Care: Body Mass Index Increases the Risk of Wound-Related Complications in Colon Cancer Surgery," *American Journal of Surgery* 207, no. 1 (January 2014): 17–23. http://www.academia.edu/6329977/Obesity_outcomes_ and_quality_of_care_body_mass_index_increases_the_risk_of_wound-related_com- plications_in_colon_cancer_surgery=.

10.  Nima Khavanin, et al., "The Influence of BMI on Perioperative Morbidity Following Abdominal Hysterectomy" abstract, *American Journal of Obstetrics and Gynecology* 208, no. 6 (June 2013): 449.e1–6.

11.  Robert W. O'Rourke, et al., "Perioperative Morbidity Associated with Bariatric Surgery: An Academic Center Experience," *Archives of Surgery* 141, no. 3 (March 2006): 262–68. http://dx.doi.org/10.1001/archsurg.141.3.262.

12.  Ted D. Adams, et al., "Long-Term Mortality after Gastric Bypass Surgery," *New England Journal of Medicine* 357 (2007): 753–61. http://dx.doi.org/10.1056/ NEJMoa066603.

13. Sandra Weineland, et al., "Acceptance and Commitment Therapy for Bariatric Surgery Patients, a Pilot RCT," *Obesity Research and Clinical Practice* 6, no. 1 (January–March 2012): e1–90. http://dx.doi.org10.1016/j.orcp.2011.04.004.

14. "Obesity Facts," Centers for Disease Control and Prevention website, accessed August 5, 2016, https://www.cdc.gov/healthyschools/obesity/facts.htm.

15. S. Jay Olshansky, et al., "A Potential Decline in Life Expectancy in the United States in the 21st Century," *New England Journal of Medicine* 352 (2005): 1138–45. http://dx.doi.org/10.1056/NEJMsr043743.

16. George A. Bray, "Medical Consequences of Obesity," *Journal of Clinical Endocrinology and Metabolism* 89, no. 6 (June 2004): 2583–89. http://dx.doi.org/10.1210/jc.2004-0535.

17. Daniel S. Hsia, Sara C. Fallon, and Mary L. Brandt, "Adolescent Bariatric Surgery," *Archives of Pediatrics and Adolescent Medicine* 166, no. 8 (August 2012): 757–66.

18. Sarah E. Barlow and the Expert Committee, "Expert Committee Recommendations Regarding the Prevention, Assessment, and Treatment of Child and Adolescent Overweight and Obesity: Summary Report," *Pediatrics* 120, suppl. 4 (2007): S164–92.

19. Traci Mann, et al., "Medicare's Search for Effective Obesity Treatments: Diets Are Not the Answer," *American Psychologist* 62, no. 3 (April 2007): 220–33. http:dx.doi.org/10.1037/0003-066X.62.3.220.

20. Dianne Neumark-Sztainer, et al., "Obesity, Disordered Eating, and Eating Disorders in a Longitudinal Study of Adolescents: How Do Dieters Fare Five Years Later?" *Journal of the American Dietetic Association* 106, no. 4 (2006): 559–68. http://dx.doi.org/10.1016/j.jada.2006.01.003.

21. Allison E. Field, et al., "Relation Between Dieting and Weight Change among Preadolescents and Adolescents," *Pediatrics* 112, no. 4 (2003): 900–906.

22. William H. Dietz, et al., "Management of Obesity," 2521–33. http://dx.doi.org/10.1016/, S0140-6736(14)61748-7.

23. Linda Bacon and Lucy Aphramor, "Weight Science: Evaluating the Evidence for a Paradigm Shift," *Nutrition Journal* 10, no. 9 (2011): 1–13.

24. Tracy L. Tylka, et al., "The Weight-Inclusive versus Weight-Normative Approach to Health: Evaluating the Evidence for Prioritizing Well-Being Over Weight Loss," *Journal of Obesity* (2014): 1–18. http://dx.doi.org/10.1155/2014/983495.

25. Tracy L. Tylka, et al., "The Weight-Inclusive versus Weight-Normative Approach to Health," 6–13. http://dx.doi.org/10.1155/2014/983495.

## CHAPTER 2

1. Evelyn Tribole and Elyse Resch, *Intuitive Eating*, 3rd ed. (New York: St. Martin's Press, 2012), 110–20.

2. R. Puhl, J. L. Peterson, and J. Luedicke, "Motivating or Stigmatizing? Public Perceptions of Weight-Related Language Used by Health Providers" abstract, *International Journal of Obesity* 37 (2013): 612–19. doi: 10.1038/ijo.2012.110.

3. Tribole and Resch, *Intuitive Eating*, 3rd ed., 80.

4. Janice A. Sabin, Maddalena Marini, and Brian A. Nosek, "Implicit and Explicit Anti-Fat Bias among a Large Sample of Medical Doctors by BMI, Race/Ethnicity and Gender," ed. Richard Fielding, *PLoS One* 7, no. 11 (November 7, 2012). http://www.ncbi.nlm.nih.gov/pmc/articles/PMC3492331/.

5. Rebecca M. Puhl and Chelsea Heuer, "Obesity Stigma: Important Considerations for Public Health," *American Journal of Public Health* 100, no. 6 (June 2010): 1019–28.

## CHAPTER 3

1. Evelyn Tribole, "Warning: Dieting Increases Your Risk of Gaining More Weight (An Update)," 2012, accessed October 27, 2015, https://www.intuitiveeating.com/content/warning-dieting-increases-your-risk-gaining-more-weight-update.

2. Tracy L. Tylka, et al., "The Weight-Inclusive versus Weight-Normative Approach to Health: Evaluating the Evidence for Prioritizing Well-Being Over Weight Loss," *Journal of Obesity* (2014): 1–18, article ID 983495. doi: http://dx.doi.org.10.1155/2014/983495.

3. Abdul G. Dulloo and Jean-Pierre Montani, "Pathways from Dieting to Weight Regain, to Obesity and to the Metabolic Syndrome: An Overview," *Obesity Reviews* 16, Suppl. 1 (February 2015): 1–6. doi:10.1111/obr.12250.

4. Abdul G. Dulloo, Jean Jacquet, and Jean-Pierre Montani, "Pathways from Weight Fluctuations to Metabolic Diseases: Focus on Maladaptive Thermogenesis During Catch-up Fat," *International Journal of Obesity and Related Metabolic Disorders* 26, Suppl. 2 (2002): S46–57.

5. Tylka, et al., "The Weight-Inclusive versus Weight-Normative Approach to Health," 1–18.

6. Traci Mann, *Secrets from the Eating Lab: The Science of Weight Loss, the Myth of Willpower, and Why You Should Never Diet Again* (New York: HarperCollins, 2015), x, 15–65.

7. Traci Mann, et al., "Medicare's Search for Effective Obesity Treatments: Diets Are Not the Answer," *American Psychologist* 62, no. 3 (April 2007): 220–33. http://dx.doi.org/10.1037/0003-066X.62.3.220.

8. "Diet" definition, Google Search, accessed October 17, 2015, https://www.google.com/?gws_rd=ssl#q=diet+definition.

9. Jennifer Taitz, *End Emotional Eating: Using Dialectical Behavioral Therapy Skills to Cope with Difficult Emotions and Develop a Healthy Relationship to Food* (Oakland: New Harbinger Publications, 2012), 15.

10. Michael D. Jensen, et al., "2013 AHA/ACC/TOS Guideline for the Management of Overweight and Obesity in Adults (Practice Guideline)," *Journal of the American College of Cardiology* 63, no. 25, table 4 (2014). http://dx.doi.org/10.1016/j.jacc.2013.11.004.

11. Jensen, et al., "2013 AHA/ACC/TOS Guideline for the Management of Overweight and Obesity in Adults (Practice Guideline)," http://dx.doi.org/ 10.1016/j.jacc.2013.11.004.

12. Linda Bacon, *Health at Every Size: The Surprising Truth about Your Weight* (Dallas: BenBella Books, 2008), 141.

13. Geoff Williams, "The Heavy Price of Losing Weight," *U.S. News and World Report*, January 2, 2013, accessed November 5, 2015, http://money.usnews.com/money/personal-finance/articles/2013/01/02/the-heavy-price-of-losing-weight.

14. Bacon, *Health at Every Size*, 164.

15. Michael R. Lowe, et al., "Dieting and Restrained Eating as Prospective Predictors of Weight Gain," *Frontiers in Psychology* 4, no. 557 (September 2013): 1–7.

16. Tylka, et al., "The Weight-Inclusive versus Weight-Normative Approach to Health," 5.

17. Bacon, *Health at Every Size*, 63.

18. Mann, *Secrets from the Eating Lab*, 15.

19. Mann, et al., "Medicare's Search for Effective Obesity Treatments," 228.

20. Mann, et al., "Medicare's Search for Effective Obesity Treatments," 224.

21. Mann, et al., "Medicare's Search for Effective Obesity Treatments," 230.

22. Bacon, *Health at Every Size*, 142.

23. Priya Sumithran and Joseph Proietto, "The Defence of Body Weight: A Physiological Basis for Weight Re-Gain After Weight Loss," *Clinical Science* 124, no. 4 (February 2013): 231–41.

24. Priya Sumithran, et al., "Long-Term Persistence of Hormonal Adaptations to Weight Loss," *New England Journal of Medicine* 365, no. 17 (October 27, 2011): 1597–604. http://dx.doi.org/10.1056/NEJMoa1105816.

25. Mann, *Secrets from the Eating Lab*, 22–23.

26. Mann, *Secrets from the Eating Lab*, 21–24.

27. Abdul G. Dulloo, Jean Jacquet, and Jean-Pierre Montani, "How Dieting Makes Some Fatter: From a Perspective of Human Body Composition Autoregulation," *Proceedings of the Nutrition Society* 71, no. 3 (August 2012): 379–89.

28. Mann, *Secrets from the Eating Lab*, 22–23.

29. Sumithran and Proietto, "The Defence of Body Weight," 231–41.

30. Sumithran and Proietto, "The Defence of Body Weight," 231–41.

31. Dulloo, Jacquet, and Montani, "Pathways from Weight Fluctuations to Metabolic Diseases," S46–57.

32. Jean-Pierre Montani, Yves Schutz, and Abdul G. Dulloo, "Dieting and Weight Cycling as Risk Factors for Cardiometabolic Diseases: Who Is Really at Risk?" abstract, *Obesity Reviews* 16, Suppl. 1 (February 2015): 7–18. http://dx.doi.org/10.1111/obr.12251.

33. Evelyn Tribole and Elyse Resch, *Intuitive Eating: A Revolutionary Program that Works* (New York: St. Martin's Griffin, 2012), 47–49.

34. Bacon, *Health at Every Size*, 47.

35. Bacon, *Health at Every Size*, 48.

36. Bacon, *Health at Every Size*, 141.

37. Bacon, *Health at Every Size*, 54.

38. Tribole, "Warning: Dieting Increases Your Risk of Gaining More Weight (An Update)," 2012, https://www.intuitiveeating.com/content/warning-dieting-increases-your-risk-gaining-more-weight-update.

39. Linda Bacon and Lucy Aphramor, "Weight Science: Evaluating the Evidence for a Paradigm Shift," *Nutrition Journal* 10 (2011): 5.

40. Mann, et al., "Medicare's Search for Effective Obesity Treatments: Diets Are Not the Answer," 220–33.

41. Bacon and Aphramor, "Weight Science: Evaluating the Evidence for a Paradigm Shift," 4.

42. A. Janet Tomiyama, et al., "Low Calorie Dieting Increases Cortisol," *Psychosomatic Medicine* 72, no. 4 (May 2010): 357–64. http:// dx.doi.org/10.1097/PSY.0b013e3181d9523c.

43. Mann, *Secrets from the Eating Lab*, 58.

44. Gina Kolata, *Rethinking Thin: The New Science of Weight Loss—and the Myths and Realities of Dieting* (New York: Picador, Farrar, Straus, and Giroux, 2007), 107–10.

45. Mann, *Secrets from the Eating Lab*, 24–25.

46. Mann, *Secrets from the Eating Lab*, 57.

47. Mann, *Secrets from the Eating Lab*, 57.

48. Karen R. Koenig, *The Rules of Normal Eating: A Commonsense Approach for Dieters, Overeaters, Undereaters, Emotional Eaters, and Everyone In Between!* (Carlsbad, CA: Gürze Books, 2005), 20.

49. Mann, *Secrets from the Eating Lab*, 8–10.

50. Tribole and Resch, *Intuitive Eating*, 52.

51. Tylka, et al., "The Weight-Inclusive versus Weight-Normative Approach to Health," 1–18.

52. Tribole and Resch, *Intuitive Eating*, 164–65.

53. Karen R. Koenig, LCSW, M.Ed., *Starting Monday: Seven Keys to a Permanent, Positive Relationship with Food* (Carlsbad: Gürze Books, 2013).

## CHAPTER 4

1. American Psychiatric Association, ed., *Diagnostic and Statistical Manual of Mental Disorders*, 5th ed. (Washington, DC: American Psychiatric Association, 2013), 339.

2. American Psychiatric Association, ed., *DSM-5*, 345.

3.  American Psychiatric Association, ed., *DSM-5*, 350–51.

4.  Ginger Nicol, "Hormones and Binge Eating Disorder," *Eating Disorder Hope*, October 2015, accessed October 1, 2015, http://www.eatingdisorderhope.com/information/binge-eating-disorder/bed-research-what-do-we-know/hormones-binge-eating-disorder.

5.  B. T. Walsh, D. E. Wilfley, and J. I. Hudson, *Binge Eating Disorder: Progress in Understanding and Treatment* (West Wayne, NJ: Health Learning Systems, 2003), 1–14.

6.  Walsh, et al., *Binge Eating Disorder*, 1–14.

7.  Walsh, et al., *Binge Eating Disorder*, 1–14.

8.  American Psychiatric Association, ed., *DSM-5*, 354.

9.  Linda Bacon, *Health at Every Size: The Surprising Truth about Your Weight* (Dallas: BenBella Books, 2008), 37–41.

10.  American Psychiatric Association, ed., *DSM-5*, 354.

11.  American Psychiatric Association, ed., *DSM-5*, 772.

12.  Zahra Jafari, Siamak Khodarahimi, and Ali Rasti, "Sexual Self-esteem and Perfectionism in Women with and Without Overweight," *Women and Therapy* 39, no. 1–2 (2016): 235–53. doi: 10.1080/02703149.2016.1116875.

13.  Daniel H. Pink, *Drive: The Surprising Truth about What Motivates Us* (New York: Riverhead Books, 2011).

14.  Karen R. Koenig, *Nice Girls Finish Fat: Put Yourself First and Change Your Eating Forever* (New York: Fireside/Simon & Schuster, 2009), 175.

15.  J. Lillis and R. R. Wing, "The Role of Avoidance-based Coping in the Psychosocial Functioning of Weight Loss Treatment-seeking Adults," *Obesity and Science Practice*, September 9, 2015, accessed October 3, 2015, http://onlinelibrary.wiley.com/doi/10.1002/osp4.1/full.

16.  American Psychiatric Association, ed., *DSM-5*, 645.

17.  International Association of Eating Disorder Professionals, "Swedish Researchers: Better Understanding of Personality Could Improve Outcome," *Eating Disorders Review* 26, no. 3 (May/June 2015), accessed September 27, 2015, http://eatingdisordersreview.com/nl/nl_edr_26_3_3.html.

18. American Psychiatric Association, ed., *DSM-5*, 663.

19. Nancy Staycer, "Co-occurring Borderline Personality Disorder and Eating Disorders," *Eating Disorder Hope*, accessed November 28, 2015, http://www.eating-disorderhope.com/treatment-for-eating-disorders/co-occurring-dual-diagnosis/trauma-ptsd/co-occurring-borderline-personality-disorder-and-eating-disorders.

20. "Symptoms of Borderline Personality Disorder," Silver Hill Hospital, accessed October 2, 2015, https://www.silverhillhospital.org/about-silver-hill/blog/july-2015-(1)/what-is-borderline-personality-disorder.

21. Carmen Keller and Michael Siegrist, "Does Personality Influence Eating Styles and Food Choices? Direct and Indirect Effects," *Appetite* 84 (January 2015): 128–38, retrieved April 2, 2016, http://www.mdlinx.com/nursing/medical-news-article/2014/11/19/big-five-personality-restrained-eating-emotional/5690973/.

22. American Psychiatric Association, ed., *DSM-5*, 673.

23. American Psychiatric Association, ed., *DSM-5*, 675.

24. "Obesity and Depression," *ConscienHealth*, accessed September 27, 2015, http://conscienhealth.org/2015/03/obesity-and-depression-co-conspirators/.

25. "Trauma & PTSD Signs, Symptoms, Effects & Risk Factors," Timberline Knolls, accessed September 20, 2015, http://www.timberlineknolls.com/trauma/signs-effects/.

26. Glenn Waller, Emma Corstorphine, and Victoria Mountford, "The Role of Emotional Abuse in the Eating Disorders: Implications for Treatment," *Eating Disorders: The Journal of Treatment and Prevention* 15, no. 4 (2007): 317–31, accessed September 27, 2015, http://www.tandfonline.com/doi/abs/10.1080/10640260701454337?src=recsys.

27. Mary Sykes Wylie, "Can Childhood Trauma Lead to Adult Obesity? How One Study Exposed the Connection Between Early Life Abuse and Weight Gain," Psychotherapy Networker, September 24, 2015, accessed September 30, 2015, https://www.psychotherapynetworker.org/blog/details/641/can-childhood-trauma-lead-to-adult-obesity.

28. Wylie, "Can Childhood Trauma Lead to Adult Obesity? How One Study Exposed the Connection Between Early Life Abuse and Weight Gain," https://www.

psychotherapynetworker.org/blog/details/641/can-childhood-trauma-lead-to-adult-obesity.

29. "Trauma and Eating Disorders," National Eating Disorders Association, accessed September 19, 2015, https://www.nationaleatingdisorders.org/sites/default/files/ResourceHandouts/TraumaandEatingDisorders.pdf.

30. Barbara Brody, "The Link Between Trauma and Binge Eating," reviewed by Joseph Goldberg, WebMD, accessed September 19, 2015, http://www.webmd.com/mental-health/eating-disorders/binge-eating-disorder/features/ptsd-binge-eating.

31. Brody, "The Link Between Trauma and Binge Eating."

32. Brody, "The Link Between Trauma and Binge Eating."

33. M. Alexis Kennedy, et al., "The Role of Childhood Emotional Abuse in Disordered Eating," *Journal of Emotional Abuse* 7, no. 1 (2007): 17–36, accessed September 27, 2015, http://www.tandfonline.com/doi/abs/10.1300/J135v07n01_02?src=recsys.

34. M. Matos, et al., "Eating Disorders: When Social Rank Perceptions are Shaped by Early Shame Experiences," *Psychology and Psychotherapy* 88, no. 1 (March 2015): 38–53, accessed February 25, 2015, http://dx.doi.org/10.1111/papt.12027.

## CHAPTER 5

1. Stephanie L. Fitzpatrick, et al., "An Evidence-based Guide for Obesity Treatment in Primary Care," *American Journal of Medicine*, accessed September 27, 2015, http://dx.doi.org/10.1016/j.amjmed.2015.07.015.

2. Gordon Cochrane, "Role for a Sense of Self-worth in Weight-loss Treatments," *Canadian Family Physician*, accessed September 27, 2015, http://www.ncbi.nlm.nih.gov/pmc/articles/PMC2294089/.

3. Cochrane, "Role for a Sense of Self-worth in Weight-loss Treatments," http://www.ncbi.nlm.nih.gov/pmc/articles/PMC2294089/.

4. Cochrane, "Role for a Sense of Self-worth in Weight-loss Treatments," http://www.ncbi.nlm.nih.gov/pmc/articles/PMC2294089/.

5. "What is CBT?" Beck Institute, accessed September 15, 2015, http://www.beckinstitute.org/history-of-cbt/.

6. Karen R. Koenig, *Starting Monday: Seven Keys to a Permanent, Positive Relationship with Food* (Carlsbad, CA: Gürze Books, 2013), 16.

7. Cochrane, "Role for a Sense of Self-worth in Weight-loss Treatments," http://
www.ncbi.nlm.nih.gov/pmc/articles/PMC2294089/.

8. Lydia Saad, "To Lose Weight, Americans Rely More on Dieting than Exercise,"
*Wellbeing*, accessed October 8, 2015, http://www.gallup.com/poll/150986/lose-
weight-americans-rely-dieting-exercise.aspx.

9. Kirstein Weir, "Feel Like a Fraud," *American Psychological Association*, November
2013, accessed October 8, 2015, http://www.apa.org/gradpsych/2013/11/fraud.aspx.

10. Karen R. Koenig, *Outsmarting Overeating: Boost Your Life Skills, End Your Food
Problems* (Novato, CA: New World Library, 2015), 3.

11. Koenig, *Outsmarting Overeating*, 3.

12. Amanda C. Crockett, Samantha K. Myhre, and Paul D. Rokke, "Boredom Proneness and Emotion Regulation Predict Emotional Eating," *Journal of Health Psychology*,
accessed September 27, 2015, http://hpq.sagepub.com/content/20/5/670.abstract.

13. Belinda Luscombe, "10 Questions with Brené Brown," *Time*, September 21,
2015, 88.

14. Crockett, Myhre, and Rokke, "Boredom Proneness and Emotion Regulation
Predict Emotional Eating," http://hpq.sagepub.com/content/20/5/670.abstract.

15. Daniel Goleman, *Emotional Intelligence: Why It Can Matter More than IQ*, 2005
ed. (New York: Bantam Dell, 2005), 55.

16. Goleman, *Emotional Intelligence*, 246–49. Citing Gloria R. Leon, Jayne
A. Fulkerson, Cheryl L. Perry, and Robert Cudeck, "Personality and Behavioral
Vulnerabilities Associated with Risk Status for Eating Disorders in Adolescent Girls,"
*Journal of Abnormal Psychology* 102, no. 3 (August 1993): 438–44. http://dx.doi.org/
10.1037/0021-843x.102.3.438.

17. Cochrane, "Role for a Sense of Self-worth in Weight-loss Treatments," http://
www.ncbi.nlm.nih.gov/pmc/articles/PMC2294089/.

18. Stan Davis, "The Truth about Bullying: How Therapists Can Help Harassed
Kids," *Psychotherapy Networker* (September/October 2012): 20; Carol Dweck,
*Mindset: The New Psychology of Success* (New York: Ballantine Books, 2008), 15–54.

19. Karen R. Koenig, *The Rules of "Normal" Eating: A Commonsense Approach
for Dieters, Overeaters, Undereaters, Emotional Eaters, and Everyone in Between!*
(Carlsbad, CA: Gürze Books, 2005), 20.

## CHAPTER 6

1. Christine Russell, "Doctors, Practice What You Preach," *Atlantic*, June 12, 2012, accessed March 12, 2016, http://www.theatlantic.com/health/archive/2012/06/doctors-practice-what-you-preach/258379/.

2. Miranda Prynne, "Overweight Doctors and Nurses Told to Slim Down by NHS Chief," *Telegraph*, July 30, 2014, accessed March 12, 2016, http://www.telegraph.co.uk/news/nhs/10999437/Overweight-doctors-and-nurses-told-to-slim-down-by-NHS-chief.html.

3. Olivia Katrandjian, "Study Finds 55 Percent of Nurses are Overweight or Obese," *ABC News*, January 30, 2012, accessed March 12, 2016, http://abcnews.go.com/Health/study-finds-55-percent-nurses-overweight-obese/story?id=15472375.

4. Katrandjian, "Study Finds 55 Percent of Nurses are Overweight or Obese," accessed March 12, 2016, http://abcnews.go.com/Health/study-finds-55-percent-nurses-overweight-obese/story?id=15472375.

5. Susan Trossman, "An Issue of Weight: Calling All Nurses to Get Healthy and Reverse a Trend," *American Nurse*, March 1, 2013, accessed March 24, 2016, http://www.theamericannurse.org/index.php/2013/03/01/an-issue-of-weight/.

6. John F. Dovidio, Kerry Kawakami, and Kelly R. Beach, ch. 9 of *Blackwell Handbook of Social Psychology: Intergroup Processes*, ed. Rupert Brown and Sam Gertner (Malden, MA: Blackwell Publishing, 2003), 175.

7. Theodore K. Kyle, Diana M. Thomas, Andrada E. Ivanescu, Joseph Hadglowski, and Rebecca M. Puhl, "Fat Shaming Is Down, But Weigh Bias Persists," *ConscienHealth*, November 6, 2015, accessed November 13, 2015, http://conscienhealth.org/2015/11/fat-shaming-is-down-but-weight-bias-persists/.

8. B. A. Teachman and K. D. Brownell, "Implicit Anti-Fat Bias among Health Professionals: Is Anyone Immune?" *International Journal of Obesity* 25, no. 10 (October 2001), http://psycnet.apa.org/psycinfo/2009-02133-002.

9. Tara Parker-Pope, The Well Column, "Are Doctors Nicer to Thinner Patients?" April 29, 2013, accessed March 12, 2016, http://well.blogs.nytimes.com/2013/04/29/overweight-patients-face-bias/?_r=0.

10. Janice A. Sabin, Maddalena Marini, and Brian A. Nosek, "Implicit and Explicit Anti-Fat Bias among a Large Sample of Medical Doctors by BMI, Race/Ethnicity and Gender," ed. Richard Fielding, *PLoS One* 7, no. 11 (November 7, 2012), http://www.ncbi.nlm.nih.gov/pmc/articles/PMC3492331/.

11. D. Q. Zhu, I. J. Norman, and A. E. White, "The Relationship Between Doctors' and Nurses' Own Weight Status and Their Weight Management Practices: A Systematic Review," *Obesity Reviews*, March 2, 2011, accessed March 12, 2016, http://onlinelibrary.wiley.com/doi/10.1111/j.1467-789X.2010.00821.x/abstract;jsessio nid=9662CC82A4E0826FB69BBBB5E7BA86AC.f03t04?userIsAuthenticated=false&d eniedAccessCustomisedMessage=.

12. Rebecca M. Puhl and Chelsea A. Heuer, "Obesity Stigma: Important Considerations for Public Health," *American Journal of Public Health* 100, no. 6 (June 2010): 1019–28, http://www.gatherthepeople.org/Downloads/OBESITY_STIGMA.pdf.

13. Puhl and Heuer, "Obesity Stigma: Important Considerations for Public Health," 1019–28, http://www.gatherthepeople.org/Downloads/OBESITY_STIGMA.pdf.

14. Puhl and Heuer, "Obesity Stigma: Important Considerations for Public Health," 1019–28, http://www.gatherthepeople.org/Downloads/OBESITY_STIGMA.pdf.

15. Jennifer Frank, "Overweight Doctors and Challenges of Staying Healthy," Physicians Practice, April 2, 2013, accessed March 12, 2016, http://www.physicianspractice.com/blog/overweight-doctors-and-challenges-staying-healthy.

16. Genevra Pittman, "Patients Often Biased against Fat Doctors, Too," Reuters, April 12, 2013, accessed March 12, 2016, http://www.reuters.com/article/2013/04/12/us-patients-fat-doctors-idUSBRE93B0S820130412.

17. Nancy Shute, "Fat Doctors Make Fat Patients Feel Better, and Worse," NPR, June 5, 2013, accessed March 12, 2016, http://www.npr.org/sections/health-shots/2013/06/05/188920874/fat-doctors-make-fat-patients-feel-better-and-worse.

18. Shute, "Fat Doctors Make Fat Patients Feel Better, and Worse," http://www.npr.org/sections/health-shots/2013/06/05/188920874/fat-doctors-make-fat-patients-feel-better-and-worse.

19. Margaret McCartney, "Fat Doctors are Patients, Too," *British Medical Journal* 349 (November 10, 2014), http://dx.doi.org/10.1136/bmj.g6464.

20. Edward Everett Hale, "I Am Only One, but Still I Am One. I Cannot Do . . ." Goodreads, accessed November 14, 2015, http://www.goodreads.com/quotes/14381-i-am-only-one-but-still-i-am-one-i.

21. Jeanne M. Ferrante, KelliAnn Seaman, Alicja Bator, Pamela Ohman-Strickland, Daniel Gundersen, Lynn Clemow, and Rebecca Puhl, "Impact of Perceived Weight Stigma among Underserved Women on Doctor-Patient Relationships," *Obesity Science and Practice*, accessed March 18, 2016, http://dx.doi.org/10.1002/osp4.40.

22. Kristin Neff, "The 5 Myths of Self-Compassion: What Keeps Us from Being Kinder to Ourselves?" *Psychotherapy Networker* 39, no. 5 (September/October 2015): 31–35, 47.

23. Tracy L. Tylka, et al., "The Weight-Inclusive versus Weight-Normative Approach to Health: Evaluating the Evidence for Prioritizing Well-Being Over Weight Loss," *Journal of Obesity* (2014): 1–18, article ID 983495. doi: http://dx.doi.org.10.1155/2014/983495.

24. Karen R. Koenig, *What Every Therapist Needs to Know about Treating Eating and Weight Issues* (New York: W.W. Norton & Co., 2008), 185.

**CHAPTER 7**

1. Linda Bacon and Lucy Aphramor, *Body Respect: What Conventional Health Books Get Wrong, Leave Out, and Just Plain Fail to Understand about Weight* (Dallas: BenBella Books, 2014), 8.

2. Vaughn W. Barrya, et al., "Fitness vs. Fatness on All-Cause Mortality: A Meta-Analysis," *Progress in Cardiovascular Diseases* 56, no. 4 (2014): 382–90. From Bacon and Aphramor, *Body Respect*, 17.

3. J. P. Montani, et al., "Weight Cycling During Growth and Beyond as a Risk Factor for Later Cardiovascular Diseases: The Repeated Overshoot Theory," *International Journal of Obesity (London)* 30, suppl. 4 (December 2006): S58–66.

4. E. Louise Thomas, et al., "The Missing Risk: MRI and MRS Phenotyping of Abdominal Adiposity and Ectopic Fat," *Obesity* 20 (2012): 76–87.

5. "Abdominal Fat and What To Do about It," Harvard Health Publications, accessed July 28, 2016, http://www.health.harvard.edu/staying-healthy/abdominal-fat-and-what-to-do-about-it.

6. Carl J. Lavie, *The Obesity Paradox: When Thinner Means Sicker and Heavier Means Healthier* (New York: Hudson Street Press, 2014), 190.

7. Lavie, *The Obesity Paradox*, 155.

8. Linda Bacon, *Health at Every Size: The Surprising Truth about Your Weight* (Dallas: BenBella Books, 2008), 141.

9. Mann, *Secrets from the Eating Lab*, 64.

10. Jennifer Taitz, *End Emotional Eating: Using Dialectical Behavioral Therapy Skills to Cope with Difficult Emotions and Develop a Healthy Relationship to Food* (Oakland: New Harbinger Publications, 2012), 3–4.

11.  Elizabeth P. Frates and Margaret Moore, "Health and Wellness Coaching Skills for Lasting Change," in *Lifestyle Medicine*, 2nd ed., ed. J. M. Rippe (New York: CRC Press, 2013), 343–60.

12.  Margaret Moore and Bob Tschannen-Moran, *Coaching Psychology Manual* (Philadelphia: Wolters Kluwer, 2010), 6.

13.  Albert Bandura, "Social Cognitive Theory of Self-Regulation," *Organizational Behavior and Human Decision Processes* 50 (1991): 248, accessed April 1, 2016, http://www.uky.edu/~eushe2/BanduraPubs/Bandura1991OBHDP.pdf.

14.  Bandura, "Social Cognitive Theory of Self-Regulation," 257, accessed April 1, 2016, http://www.uky.edu/~eushe2/BanduraPubs/Bandura1991OBHDP.pdf.

15.  Steven Stosny, Ph.D., "Self-Regulation: To Feel Better, Focus on What Is Most Important," accessed April 3, 2016, posted October 28, 2011, at https://www.psychol-ogytoday.com/blog/anger-in-the-age-entitlement/201110/self-regulation.

16.  Taitz, *End Emotional Eating*, 16.

17.  Taitz, *End Emotional Eating*, 72–73.

18.  Daniel Goleman, *Emotional Intelligence: Why It Can Matter More Than IQ* (New York: Bantam Books, 2005).

19.  Brian Tracy, *Goals: How to Get Everything You Want—Faster Than You Ever Thought Possible*, 2nd ed. (Oakland: Berrett-Koehler Publishers, 2010).

20.  Brian Tracy, *Change Your Thinking, Change Your Life: How to Unlock Your Full Potential for Success and Achievement* (New York: MJF Books, 2003), 46.

21.  Gordon Cochrane, "Role for Self-worth in Weight-loss Treatments," *Canadian Family Physician* 54 (April 2008): 543–46.

22.  Taitz, *End Emotional Eating*, 178.

23.  Taitz, *End Emotional Eating*, 186, citing C. E. Adams and M. R. Leary, "Promoting Self-compassionate Attitudes toward Eating among Restrictive and Guilty Eaters," *Journal of Social and Clinical Psychology* 26 (2007): 1120–44.

24.  Kristin Neff, *Self-Compassion: The Proven Power of Being Kind to Yourself* (New York: William Morrow, 2011), 122.

25.  Karen R. Koenig, *The Food & Feelings Workbook: A Full Course Meal on Emotional Health* (Carlsbad, CA: Gürze Books, 2007), 21.

26.  Taitz, *End Emotional Eating*, 3–4.

27. Taitz, *End Emotional Eating*, 5.

28. Taitz, *End Emotional Eating*, 183.

29. Neff, *Self-Compassion*, 109.

30. Neff, *Self-Compassion*, 177.

31. The Principles of Mindful Eating, accessed July 28, 2016, http://thecenterfor-mindfuleating.org/Principles-Mindful-Eating.

32. Tribole and Resch, *Intuitive Eating*, 3rd ed., 35–37.

33. Nina Van Dyke and Eric J. Drinkwater, "Relationships Between Intuitive Eating and Health Indicators: Literature Review," *Public Health Nutrition* 17, no. 8 (2013): 1757–66.

34. Margaret Moore, Erika Jackson, and Bob Tschannen-Moran, *Coaching Psychology Manual*, 2nd ed. (Philadelphia: Wolters Kluwer, 2016), 65–75.

35. Tracy, "Visualize Your Goals Continually," in *Goals*, 237–51.

36. Moore, Jackson, and Tschannen-Moran, *Coaching Psychology Manual*, 2nd ed., 129–33.

37. Tracy, "Clarify Your Values," in *Goals*, 29–39.

38. Stephen Rollnick, William R. Miller, and Christopher C. Butler, *Motivational Interviewing in Health Care: Helping Patients Change Behavior* (New York: The Guilford Press, 2008), 9.

39. Rollnick, Miller, and Butler, *Motivational Interviewing in Health Care*, 40–41.

40. Moore, Jackson, and Tschannen-Moran, *Coaching Psychology Manual*, 2nd ed., 82.

41. Rollnick, Miller, and Butler, *Motivational Interviewing in Health Care*, 40–41.

42. Dennis Waitley, *The Psychology of Success*, 6th ed. (New York: McGraw Hill Education, 2016), 4.

43. Waitley, *The Psychology of Success*, 6th ed., 4–8.

44. Moore, Jackson, and Tschannen-Moran, *Coaching Psychology Manual*, 2nd ed., 32.

45. Google search for persistence, accessed April 1, 2016, https://www.google.com/search?q=persistencee&ie=utf-8&oe=utf-8#q=persistence.

46. Moore, Jackson, and Tschannen-Moran, *Coaching Psychology Manual*, 2nd ed., 86.

47. "Habits: How They Form and How to Break Them," NPR, interview with journalist Charles Duhigg, author of *The Power of Habit: Why We Do What We Do In Life and In Business* (New York: Random House, 2012), March 5, 2012, accessed March 30, 2016, http://www.npr.org/2012/03/05/147192599/ habits-how-they-form-and-how-to-break-them.

48. Carol A. Seger and Brian J. Spiering, "A Critical Review of Habit Learning and the Basil Ganglia," *Frontiers In Systems Neuroscience* 4, no. 66 (2011): 1–9, accessed March 30, 2016, http://dx.doi.org/10.3389/fnsys.2011.00066.

49. Benjamin Gardner, Phillippa Lally, and Jane Wardle, "Making Health Habitual: The Psychology of 'Habit Formation' and General Practice," *British Journal of General Practice* 62 (December 2012): 663–66. http://dx.doi.org/10.3399/ bjgp12X659466.

## CHAPTER 8

1. Linda Bacon, Ph.D., *Health at Every Size: The Surprising Truth about Your Weight* (Dallas: BenBella Books, 2008), 141.

2. Abdul G. Dulloo, Jean Jacquet, and Jean-Pierre Montani, "Pathways from Weight Fluctuations to Metabolic Diseases: Focus on Maladaptive Thermogenesis During Catch-up Fat," *International Journal of Obesity and Related Metabolic Disorders* 26, Suppl. 2 (2002): S46–57.

3. Kristin Neff, *Self Compassion: The Proven Power of Being Kind to Yourself* (New York: William Morrow, 2011), 109.

4. Tracy L. Tylka, et al., "The Weight-Inclusive Versus Weight-Normative Approach to Health: Evaluating the Evidence for Prioritizing Well-Being Over Weight Loss," *Journal of Obesity* (2014): 1–18.

5. Evelyn Tribole and Elyse Resch, *Intuitive Eating*, 3rd ed. (New York: St. Martin's Press, 2005), 235–38.

6. Tribole and Resch, *Intuitive Eating*, 3rd ed.

7. "Progress on Obesity," Centers for Disease Control and Prevention, accessed March 21, 2016, http://www.cdc.gov/vitalsigns/childhoodobesity/.

8. Tribole and Resch, *Intuitive Eating*, 3rd ed., 230.

9. Dianne Neumark-Sztainer, et al., "Dieting and Disordered Eating Behaviors from Adolescence to Young Adulthood: Findings from a 10-Year Longitudinal Study,"

*Journal of the American Dietetic Association* 111 (2011): 1004–11. doi: 10.1016/
j.jada.2011.04.012.

10. Evelyn Tribole, "Warning: Dieting Increases Your Risk of Gaining More Weight
(An Update)," 2012, accessed September 12, 2015, https://www.intuitiveeating.com/
content/warning-dieting-increases-your-risk-gaining-more-weight-update.

11. Tylka, et al., "The Weight-Inclusive Versus Weight-Normative Approach to
Health," 6.

12. Tylka, et al., "The Weight-Inclusive Versus Weight-Normative Approach to
Health," 6.

13. Tylka, et al., "The Weight-Inclusive Versus Weight-Normative Approach to
Health," 6.

14. Tracy L. Tylka and Nichole Wood-Barcalow, "What Is and What Is Not Positive Body Image? Conceptual Foundations and Construct Definition," *Body Image*
(2015), http://dx.doi.org/10.1016/j.bodyim.2015.04.001.

15. Linda Bacon and Lucy Aphramor, "Weight Science: Evaluating the Evidence for
a Paradigm Shift," *Nutrition Journal* 10, no. 9 (2011): 5.

16. Tracy L. Tylka and Nichole Wood-Barcalow, "The Body Appreciation Scale-2:
Item Refinement and Psychometric Evaluation," *Body Image* 12 (January 2015):
53–67. http://www.sciencedirect.com/science/article/pii/S1740144514001314.

17. Tylka, et al., "The Weight-Inclusive Versus Weight-Normative Approach to
Health," 1–18.

18. Bacon, *Health at Every Size.*

19. Tylka, et al., "The Weight-Inclusive versus Weight-Normative Approach to
Health," 10.

20. Tribole and Resch, *Intuitive Eating*, 3rd ed., 239–40.

21. Nina Van Dyke and Eric J Drinkwater, "Relationships Between Intuitive Eating
and Health Indicators: Literature Review," *Public Health Nutrition* 17, no. 8 (August
2014): 1757–66.

22. Tracy L. Tylka and Ashley M. Kroon Van Diest, "The Intuitive Eating Scale–2:
Item Refinement and Psychometric Evaluation with College Women and Men," *Journal
of Counseling Psychology* 60, no. 1 (January 2013): 137–53. http://dx.doi.org/10.1037/
a0030893, accessed at http://www.ncbi.nlm.nih.gov/pubmed/23356469 on April 3, 2016.

23. Margaret Moore, Erika Jackson, and Bob Tschannen-Moran, *Coaching Psychology Manual*, 2nd ed. (Philadelphia: Wolters Kluwer, 2016), 58.

24. William R. Miller, Stephen Rollnick, and Christopher C. Butler, *Motivational Interviewing in Health Care: Helping Patients Change Behavior* (New York: The Guilford Press, 2008), 98.

25. Center for Building a Culture of Empathy, Wikipedia, accessed April 1, 2016 at http://cultureofempathy.com/projects/Empathy-Movement/References/Reflective-Listening.htm.

26. Margaret Moore and Bob Tschannen-Moran, *Coaching Psychology Manual* (Philadelphia: Lippincott, Williams & Wilkins, 2010), 64–65.

27. Marshall B. Rosenberg, *Nonviolent Communication: A Language of Life*, 3rd ed. (Encinitas, CA: Puddledancer Press, 2015).

28. Moore, Jackson, and Tschannen-Moran, *Coaching Psychology Manual*, 2nd ed., 37–38.

29. Moore, Jackson, and Tschannen-Moran, *Coaching Psychology Manual*, 2nd ed., 107.

30. Neff, *Self Compassion*, 10.

31. Taitz, *End Emotional Eating*, 178–83.

32. Claire E. Adams and Mark R. Leary, "Promoting Self-compassionate Attitudes toward Eating among Restrictive and Guilty Eaters," *Journal of Social and Clinical Psychology* 26, no. 10 (2007): 1120–44, as cited in Taitz, 186.

33. Neff, *Self Compassion*, 170.

34. Neff, *Self Compassion*, 182.

35. Neff, *Self Compassion*, 166.

36. Neff, *Self Compassion*, 162.

37. Tylka, et al., "The Weight-Inclusive Versus Weight-Normative Approach to Health," 1–18.

38. Kelley Raab, "Mindfulness, Self-Compassion, and Empathy among Health Care Professionals: A Review of the Literature," *Journal of Health Care Chaplaincy* 20, no. 3 (2014): 95–108. http://dx.doi.org/10.1080/08854726.2014.913876.

39. Emma M. Seppala, et al., "Loving-Kindness Meditation: A Tool to Improve Healthcare Provider Compassion, Resilience, and Patient Care," *Journal of Compassionate Health Care* 1 (2014): 5. doi: 10.1186/s40639-014-0005-9.

40. Tylka, et al., "The Weight-Inclusive Versus Weight-Normative Approach to Health," 13.

41. Miller, Rollnick, and Butler, *Motivational Interviewing in Health Care*, 5.

42. Margaret Moore and Bob Tschannen-Moran, *Coaching Psychology Manual* (Philadelphia: Wolters Kluwer, 2010), 64.

43. Ellen Glovsky, ed., *Wellness, Not Weight: Health at Every Size and Motivational Interviewing* (San Diego, CA: Cognella Academic Publishing, 2014), xiv.

44. Miller, Rollnick, and Butler, *Motivational Interviewing in Health Care*, 66.

45. David Cooperrider and Diana Whitney, *Appreciative Inquiry: A Positive Revolution in Change* (San Francisco: Berrett-Koehler, 2005).

46. Moore, Jackson, and Tschannen-Moran, *Coaching Psychology Manual*, 2nd ed., 72.

47. J. O. Prochaska and C. C. DiClemente, "Stages and Process of Self-Change of Smoking: Toward an Integrative Model of Change," *Journal of Consulting and Clinical Psychology* 51, no. 3 (1983): 390–95.

48. Moore, Jackson, and Tschannen-Moran, *Coaching Psychology Manual*, 2nd ed., 93–111.

49. Moore, Jackson, and Tschannen-Moran, *Coaching Psychology Manual*, 2nd ed., 94–102.

50. Moore and Tschannen-Moran, *Coaching Psychology Manual*, 93–97.

51. Karen R. Koenig, LCSW, M.Ed., *Starting Monday: Seven Keys to a Permanent, Positive Relationship to Food* (Carlsbad: Gürze Books, 2013), 116–21.

52. Moore, Jackson, and Tschannen-Moran, *Coaching Psychology Manual*, 2nd ed., 133.

53. George T. Doran, "There's a S.M.A.R.T. Way to Write Management's Goals and Objectives," *Management Review* 70, no. 11 (1981): 35–36.

54. Denis Waitley, *Psychology of Success: Finding Meaning in Work and Life*, 6th ed. (New York: McGraw Hill Education, 2016), 90–93.

55. Moore, Jackson, and Tschannen-Moran, *Coaching Psychology Manual*, 2nd ed., 133.

56. Daniel Goleman, *Emotional Intelligence: Why It Can Matter More than IQ* (New York: Bantam Dell, 2005), xi, xiv, 36.

57. Linda Bacon and Lucy Aphramor, "Weight Science: Evaluating the Evidence for a Paradigm Shift," *Nutrition Journal* 10, no. 9 (2011): 1–13.

58. "Why is Lifestyle Medicine Essential to Sustainable Health and Health Care?" American College of Lifestyle Medicine, accessed March 1, 2016, http://www.lifestylemedicine.org/What-is-Lifestyle-Medicine.

59. "Why is Lifestyle Medicine Essential to Sustainable Health and Health Care?"

60. Rani Polak, Rachele M. Pojednic, and Edward M. Phillips, "Lifestyle Medicine Education," *American Journal of Lifestyle Medicine* 9, no. 5 (September 2015): 361–67. doi: 10.1177/1559827615580307.

61. ACLM President, David Katz, M.D., M.P.H., ACLM website, http://www.lifestylemedicine.org.

62. "The Lifestyle Medicine Dream Team," presented at Harvard Medical School Lifestyle Medicine Conference, June 2015, http://www.lifestylemedicine.hmscme.com/sites/lifestylemedicine.hmscme.com/files/course-info/Lifestyle%20Medicine%202015%20web_EB.pdf.

63. Polak, Pojednic, and Phillips, "Lifestyle Medicine Education," 361–67.

64. "NCCHWC Announces Launch of National Certification for Professional Health and Wellness Coaches," press release of April 30, 2015, accessed on April 10, 2016, http://www.ncchwc.org/PR043015.pdf.

65. Meg Jordan, et al., "National Training and Education Standards for Health and Wellness Coaching: The Path to National Certification," *Global Advances In Health and Medicine* 4, no. 3 (May 2015). doi: 10.7453/gahmj.2015.039.

66. Pedro J. Teixeira, et al., "Successful Behavior Change in Obesity Interventions in Adults: A Systematic Review of Self-Regulation Mediators," *BMC Medicine* 13, no. 84 (April 2015), http://dx.doi.org/10.1186/s12916-015-0323-6.

67. "What is Wellness Coaching?" Real Balance, accessed March 29, 2016, https://www.realbalance.com/what-is-wellness-coaching.

68. Tylka, et al., "The Weight-Inclusive Versus Weight-Normative Approach to Health," 1–18.

69. "American College of Lifestyle Medicine Announces Partnership with Well-coaches Corporation," PR Web, accessed March 10, 2016, http://www.prweb.com/releases/2015/11/prweb13062478.htm.

70. "American College of Lifestyle Medicine Announces Partnership with Wellcoaches Corporation," http://www.prweb.com/releases/2015/11/prweb13062478.htm.

71. "American College of Lifestyle Medicine Announces Partnership with Well-coaches Corporation."

72. David Eisenberg and Jonathan Burgess, "Nutrition Education in an Era of Global Obesity and Diabetes: Thinking Outside the Box," *Academic Medicine* 90, no. 7 (July 2015): 854–60.

73. Rani Polak, et al., "Health-Related Culinary Education: A Summary of Representative Emerging Programs for Health Professionals and Patients," *Global Advances in Health and Medicine* 5, no. 1 (2016): 61–68. doi: 10.7453/gahmj.2015.128.

74. Polak, et al., "Health-Related Culinary Education," 63–64.

75. Susie Orbach, *Fat Is a Feminist Issue: The Anti-Diet Guide for Women* (New York: Galahad Books, 1997), 99–122.

76. Dave Sabgir, Walk With a Doc, http://walkwithadoc.org/who-we-are/metrics/.

77. Bert N. Uchino, "Social Support and Health: A Review of Physiological Processes Potentially Underlying Links to Disease Outcomes," *Journal of Behavioral Medicine* 29, no. 4 (2006): 377–87, http://dx.doi.org/10.1007/s10865-006-9056-5.

78. George Latimer Apperson, *The Wordsworth Dictionary of Proverbs*, 283, accessed March 28, 2016, https://books.google.com/books?id=7PMZJqSR4sAC&lpg=PA283&dq=%22first+law+of+holes%22+Healy&pg=PA283&hl=en#v=onepage&q&f=false. Ware: Wordsworth Editions, p. 283 on Law of holes, Dennis Healey (2006).

79. Tylka, et al., "The Weight-Inclusive Versus Weight-Normative Approach to Health," 1–18.

# Bibliography

"Abdominal Fat and What to Do about It." Harvard Health Publications. Accessed July 28, 2016 at http://www.health.harvard.edu/staying-healthy/abdominal-fat-and-what-to-do-about-it.

Adams, Claire E., and Mark R. Leary. "Promoting Self-compassionate Attitudes toward Eating among Restrictive and Guilty Eaters." *Journal of Social and Clinical Psychology* 26, no. 10 (2007): 1120–44.

Adams, Kelly M., Martin Kohlmeier, and Steven H. Zeisel. "Nutrition Education in U.S. Medical Schools: Latest Update of a National Survey." *Academic Medicine* 85, no. 9 (2010): 1537–42. http://dx.doi.org/10.1097/ACM.0b013e3181eab71b.

Adams, Ted D., Richard E. Gress, Sherman C. Smith, R. Chad Halverson, Steven C. Simper, Wayne D. Rosamond, Michael J. LaMonte, Antoinette M. Stroup, and Steven C. Hunt. "Long-Term Mortality after Gastric Bypass Surgery," abstract. *New England Journal of Medicine* 357 (2007): 753–61. http://dx.doi.org/10.1056/NEJMoa066603.

"American College of Lifestyle Medicine Announces Partnership with Wellcoaches Corporation." PR Web. Accessed March 10, 2016. http://www.prweb.com/releases/2015/11/prweb13062478.htm.

American Psychiatric Association, ed. *Diagnostic and Statistical Manual of Mental Disorders.* 5th ed. Washington, DC: American Psychiatric Association, 2013.

Apperson, George Latimer. *The Wordsworth Dictionary of Proverbs*, 283. Accessed March 28, 2016. https://books.google.com/books?id=7PMZJqSR4sAC&lpg=PA28

3&dq=%22first+law+of+holes%22+Healy&pg=PA283&hl=en#v=onepage&q&f= false. Ware: Wordsworth Editions, p. 283 on Law of holes, Dennis Healey (2006).

Bacon, Linda. *Health at Every Size: The Surprising Truth about Your Weight*. Dallas: BenBella Books, 2008.

Bacon, Linda, and Lucy Aphramor. *Body Respect: What Conventional Health Books Get Wrong, Leave Out, and Just Plain Fail to Understand about Weight*. Dallas: BenBella Books, 2014.

Bacon, Linda, and Lucy Aphramor. "Weight Science: Evaluating the Evidence for a Paradigm Shift." *Nutrition Journal* 10 (2011): 1–13.

Bandura, Albert. "Self-efficacy: Toward a Unifying Theory of Behavioral Change." *Psychological Review* 84, no. 2 (1977): 191–215.

Bandura, Albert. "Social Cognitive Theory of Self-Regulation." *Organizational Behavior and Human Decision Processes* 50 (1991): 257. Accessed April 1, 2016. http://www. uky.edu/~eushe2/BanduraPubs/Bandura1991OBHDP.pdf.

Barlow, Sarah E., and the Expert Committee. "Expert Committee Recommendations Regarding the Prevention, Assessment, and Treatment of Child and Adolescent Overweight and Obesity: Summary Report." *Pediatrics* 120, suppl. 4 (2007): S164–92.

Barrya, Vaughn W., Meghan Baruth, Michael W. Beets, J. Larry Durstine, Jihong Liu, and Steven N. Blair. "Fitness vs. Fatness on All-cause Mortality: A Meta-analysis." *Progress in Cardiovascular Diseases* 56, no. 4 (2014): 382–90.

Blair, Steven N., Jessica Shaten, Kelly Brownell, Gary Collins, and Lauren Lissner. "Body Weight Change, All-cause Mortality, and Cause-specific Mortality in the Multiple Risk Factor Intervention Trial," abstract. *Annals of Internal Medicine* 119, no. 7, pt. 2 (1993): 749–57.

Bray, George A. "Medical Consequences of Obesity." *Journal of Clinical Endocrinology and Metabolism* 89, no. 6 (June 2004): 2583–89. http://dx.doi.org/10.1210/ jc.2004-0535.

Brody, Barbara. "The Link Between Trauma and Binge Eating." Reviewed by Joseph Goldberg. WebMD. Accessed September 19, 2015. http://www.webmd.com/ mental-health/eating-disorders/binge-eating-disorder/features/ptsd-binge-eating.

Center for Building a Culture of Empathy. Wikipedia. Accessed April 1, 2016. http:// cultureofempathy.com/projects/Empathy-Movement/References/Reflective-Listening.htm.

Cochrane, Gordon. "Role for a Sense of Self-worth in Weight-loss Treatments." *Canadian Family Physician* 54 (April 2008): 543–46. Accessed September 27, 2015. http://www.ncbi.nlm.nih.gov/pmc/articles/PMC2294089/.

Collins, M. E. "Body Figure Perceptions and Preferences among Pre-adolescent Children." *International Journal of Eating Disorders* 10, no. 2 (1991): 199–208.

Cooperrider, David, and Diana Whitney. *Appreciative Inquiry: A Positive Revolution in Change*. San Francisco: Berrett-Koehler, 2005.

Crockett, Amanda C., Samantha K. Myhre, and Paul D. Rokke. "Boredom Proneness and Emotion Regulation Predict Emotional Eating." *Journal of Health Psychology*. Accessed September 27, 2015. http://hpq.sagepub.com/content/20/5/670.abstract.

"Diet" definition, Google Search. Accessed October 17, 2015. https://www.google.com/?gws_rd=ssl#q=diet+definition.

Dietz, William H., Louise A. Baur, Kevin Hall, Rebecca M. Puhl, Elsie M. Taveras, Ricardo Uauy, and Peter Kopelman. "Management of Obesity: Improvement of Health-Care Training and Systems for Prevention and Care." *Lancet* 385 (2015): 2521–33. http://dx.doi.org/10.1016/, S0140-6736(14)61748-7.

Doran, George T. "There's a S.M.A.R.T. Way to Write Management's Goals and Objectives." *Management Review* 70, no. 11 (1981): 35–36.

Dovidio, John F., Kerry Kawakami, and Kelly R. Beach. Chap. 9 of *Blackwell Handbook of Social Psychology: Intergroup Processes*. Edited by Rupert Brown and Sam Gertner. Malden, MA: Blackwell Publishing, 2003.

Dulloo, Abdul G., Jean Jacquet, and Jean-Pierre Montani. "How Dieting Makes Some Fatter: From a Perspective of Human Body Composition Autoregulation." *Proceedings of the Nutrition Society* 71, no. 3 (August 2012): 379–89.

Dulloo, Abdul G., Jean Jacquet, and Jean-Pierre Montani. "Pathways from Weight Fluctuations to Metabolic Diseases: Focus on Maladaptive Thermogenesis During Catch-up Fat." *International Journal of Obesity and Related Metabolic Disorders* 26, suppl. 2 (2002): S46–57.

Dweck, Carol. *Mindset: The New Psychology of Success*. New York: Ballantine Books, 2008.

Eisenberg, David, and Jonathan Burgess. "Nutrition Education in an Era of Global Obesity and Diabetes: Thinking Outside the Box." *Academic Medicine* 90, no. 7 (July 2015): 854–60.

Ellis, Samantha, Katherine Rosenblum, Alison Miller, and Karen E. Peterson. "Meaning of the Terms 'Overweight' and 'Obese' among Low-Income Women." *Journal of Nutrition Education and Behavior* 46, no. 4 (July–August 2014): 299–303. doi:10.1016/j.jneb.2013.08.006.

Ferrante, Jeanne M., KelliAnn Seaman, Alicja Bator, Pamela Ohman-Strickland, Daniel Gundersen, Lynn Clemow, and Rebecca Puhl. "Impact of Perceived Weight Stigma among Underserved Women on Doctor-Patient Relationships." *Obesity Science and Practice.* Accessed March 18, 2016. http://dx.doi.org/10.1002/osp4.40.

Field, Allison E., S. B. Austin, C. B. Taylor, Susan Malspeis, Bernard Rosner, Helaine R. Rockett, Matthew W. Gillman, and Graham A. Colditz. "Relation Between Dieting and Weight Change among Preadolescents and Adolescents," abstract. *Pediatrics* 112, no. 4 (October 2003): 900–906.

Fitzpatrick, Stephanie L., Danielle Wischenka, Bradley M. Appelhans, Lori Robert, Monica Wang, Dawn K. Wilson, and Sherry L. Pagoto. "An Evidence-based Guide for Obesity Treatment in Primary Care." *American Journal of Medicine.* Accessed September 27, 2015. http://dx.doi.org/10.1016/j.amjmed.2015.07.015.

Frank, Jennifer. "Overweight Doctors and Challenges of Staying Healthy." *Physicians Practice,* April 2, 2013. http://www.physicianspractice.com/blog/overweight-doctors-and-challenges-staying-healthy.

Frates, Elizabeth P., and Margaret Moore. "Health and Wellness Coaching Skills for Lasting Change." In *Lifestyle Medicine,* 2nd ed. Edited by J. M. Rippe, 343–60. New York: CRC Press, 2013.

Gardner, Benjamin, Phillippa Lally, and Jane Wardle. "Making Health Habitual: The Psychology of 'Habit Formation' and General Practice." *British Journal of General Practice* 62, no. 605 (December 2012): 663–66. http://dx.doi.org/10.3399/bjgp12X659466.

Glanc, Phyllis, et al. "Challenges of Pelvic Imaging in Obese Women." *Radiographics* 32, no. 6 (2012): 1839–62. doi: 10.1148/rg.326125510.

Glovsky, Ellen, ed. *Wellness, Not Weight: Health at Every Size and Motivational Interviewing.* San Diego: Cognella Academic Publishing, 2014.

Goleman, Daniel. *Emotional Intelligence: Why it Can Matter More Than IQ.* 2005 ed. New York: Bantam Dell, 2005.

Gudzune, Kimberly A., Wendy L. Bennett, Lisa A. Cooper, and Sara N. Bleich. "Patients Who Feel Judged about Their Weight Have Lower Trust in Their Primary Care Providers." *Patient Education Counseling* 97, no. 1 (October 2014): 128–31. http://dx.doi.org/10.1015/j.pec.2014.06.019.

"Habits: How They Form and How to Break Them." NPR, interview with journalist Charles Duhigg, author of *The Power of Habit: Why We Do What We Do in Life and in Business* (New York: Random House, 2012), March 5, 2012. Accessed March 30, 2016. http://www.npr.org/2012/03/05/147192599/habits-how-they-form-and-how-to-break-them.

Hale, Edward Everett. "I Am Only One, but Still I Am One. I Cannot Do . . ." Goodreads. Accessed November 14, 2015. http://www.goodreads.com/quotes/14381-i-am-only-one-but-still-i-am-one-i.

Hsia, Daniel S., Sara C. Fallon, and Mary L. Brandt. "Adolescent Bariatric Surgery," abstract. *Archives of Pediatric and Adolescent Medicine* 166, no. 8 (August 2012): 757–66.

International Association of Eating Disorder Professionals. "Swedish Researchers: Better Understanding of Personality Could Improve Outcome." *Eating Disorders Review* 26, no. 3 (May/June 2015). Accessed September 27, 2015. http://eatingdisordersreview.com/nl/nl_edr_26_3_3.html.

"Jacobellis v. Ohio." Legal Information Institute. Accessed September 7, 2015. https://www.law.cornell.edu/supremecourt/text/378/184#writing-USSC_CR_0378_0184_ZC1.

Jafari, Zahra, Siamak Khodarahimi, and Ali Rasti. "Sexual Self-esteem and Perfectionism in Women with and Without Overweight." *Women and Therapy* 39, nos. 1–2 (2016). http://dx.doi.org/10.1080/02703149.2016.1116875.

Jensen, Michael D., Donna H. Ryan, Caroline M. Apovian, Jamy D. Ard, Anthony G. Comuzzie, Karen A. Donato, Frank B. Hu, Van S. Hubbard, John M. Jakicic, Robert F. Kushner, Catherine M. Loria, Barbara E. Millen, Cathy A. Nonas, F. Xavier Pi-Sunyer, June Stevens, Victor J. Stevens, Thomas A. Wadden, Bruce M. Wolfe, and Susan Z. Yanovski. "2013 AHA/ACC/TOS Guideline for the Management of Overweight and Obesity in Adults (Practice Guideline)." *Journal of the American College of Cardiology* 63, no. 25 (2014). http://dx.doi.org/10.1016/j.jacc.2013.11.004.

Jordan, Meg, Ruth Q. Wolever, Karen Lawson, and Margaret Moore. "National Training and Education Standards for Health and Wellness Coaching: The Path to National Certification." *Global Advances in Health and Medicine* 4, no. 3 (May 2015): 46–56. doi:10.7453/gahmj.2015.039.

Joshi, Girish P., Saravanan P. Ankichetty, Tong J. Gan, and Frances Chung. "Society for Ambulatory Anesthesia Consensus Statement on Preoperative Selection of Adult Patients with Obstructive Sleep Apnea Scheduled for Ambulatory Surgery," abstract. *Anesthesia & Analgesia Journal* 115, no. 5 (November 2012): 1060–68. http://dx.doi.org/10.1213/ANE.0b013e318269cfd7.

Katrandjian, Olivia. "Study Finds 55 Percent of Nurses are Overweight or Obese." ABC News, January 30, 2012. http://abcnews.go.com/Health/study-finds-55-percent-nurses-overweight-obese/story?id=15472375.

Keller, Carmen, and Michael Siegrist. "Does Personality Influence Eating Styles and Food Choices? Direct and Indirect Effects." *Appetite* 84 (January 2015): 128–38. Retrieved April 2, 2016. http://www.mdlinx.com/nursing/medical-news-article/2014/11/19/big-five-personality-restrained-eating-emotional/5690973/.

Kennedy, M. Alexis, Karen Ip, Joti Samra, and Boris B. Gorzalka. "The Role of Childhood Emotional Abuse in Disordered Eating." *Journal of Emotional Abuse* 7, no. 1 (2007). Accessed September 27, 2015. http://www.tandfonline.com/doi/abs/10.1300/J135v07n01_02?src=recsys.

Khavanin, Nima, Francis C. Lovecchio, Philip J. Hanwright, Elizabeth Brill, Magdy Milad, Karl Y. Bilimoria, and John Y. S. Kim. "The Influence of BMI on Perioperative Morbidity Following Abdominal Hysterectomy," abstract. *American Journal of Obstetrics and Gynecology* 208, no. 6 (June 2013): 449.e1–6.

Koenig, Karen R. *The Food & Feelings Workbook: A Full Course Meal on Emotional Health.* Carlsbad: Gürze Books, 2007.

Koenig, Karen R. *Nice Girls Finish Fat: Put Yourself First and Change Your Eating Forever.* New York: Fireside/Simon & Schuster, 2009.

Koenig, Karen R. *Outsmarting Overeating: Boost Your Life Skills, End Your Food Problems.* Novato, CA: New World Library, 2015.

Koenig, Karen R. *The Rules of "Normal" Eating: A Commonsense Approach for Dieters, Overeaters, Undereaters, Emotional Eaters, and Everyone in Between!* Carlsbad, CA: Gürze Books, 2005.

Koenig, Karen R. *Starting Monday: Seven Keys to a Permanent, Positive Relationship with Food.* Carlsbad, CA: Gürze Books, 2013.

Koenig, Karen R. *What Every Therapist Needs to Know about Treating Eating and Weight Issues.* New York: W.W. Norton & Co., 2008.

Kolata, Gina. *Rethinking Thin: The New Science of Weight Loss—and the Myths and Realities of Dieting.* New York: Picador, Farrar, Straus, and Giroux, 2007.

Kyle, Theodore K., Diana M. Thomas, Andrada E. Ivanescu, Joseph Hadglowski, and Rebecca M. Puhl. "Fat Shaming Is Down, But Weigh Bias Persists." *ConscienHealth*, November 6, 2015. Accessed November 13, 2015. http://conscienhealth.org/2015/11/fat-shaming-is-down-but-weight-bias-persists/.

Lavie, Carl J. *The Obesity Paradox: When Thinner Means Sicker and Heavier Means Healthier.* New York: Hudson Street Press, 2014.

Leon, Gloria R., Jayne A. Fulkerson, Cheryl L. Perry, and Robert Cudeck. "Personality and Behavioral Vulnerabilities Associated with Risk Status for Eating Disorders in Adolescent Girls." *Journal of Abnormal Psychology* 102, no. 3 (August 1993): 438–44. http://dx.doi.org/10.1037/0021-843x.102.3.438.

Lillis, J., and R. R. Wing. "The Role of Avoidance-Based Coping in the Psychosocial Functioning of Weight Loss Treatment-Seeking Adults." *Obesity and Science Practice*, September 9, 2015. Accessed October 3, 2015. doi:10.1002/osp4.1.

Lowe, Michael R., Sapna D. Doshi, Shawn N. Katterman, and Emily H. Feig. "Dieting and Restrained Eating as Prospective Predictors of Weight Gain." *Frontiers in Psychology* 4, no. 557 (September 2013): 1–7.

Luscombe, Belinda. "10 Questions with Brené Brown." *Time*, September 21, 2015.

Mann, Traci. *Secrets from the Eating Lab: The Science of Weight Loss, the Myth of Willpower, and Why You Should Never Diet Again.* New York: HarperCollins, 2015.

Mann, Traci, A. Janet Tomiyama, Erika Westling, Ann-Marie Lew, Barbra Samuels, and Jason Chatman. "Medicare's Search for Effective Obesity Treatments: Diets Are Not the Answer." *American Psychologist* 62, no. 3 (April 2007): 220–33. http://dx.doi.org/10.1037/0003-066X.62.3.220.

Matos, M., C. Ferreira, C. Duarte, and J. Pinto-Gouveia. "Eating Disorders: When Social Rank Perceptions are Shaped by Early Shame Experiences." *Psychology and Psychotherapy* 88, no. 1 (March 2015). Accessed February 25, 2015. http://dx.doi.org/10.1111/papt.12027.

May, Michelle. *Eat What You Love, Love What You Eat: How to Break Your Eat-Repent-Repeat Cycle.* Austin: GreenLeaf Book Group Press, 2010.

McCartney, Margaret. "Fat Doctors are Patients, Too." *British Medical Journal*, November 10, 2014. http://dx.doi.org/10.1136/bmj.g6464.

Montani, J. P., A. K. Viecelli, A. Prévot, and A. G. Dulloo. "Weight Cycling During Growth and Beyond as a Risk Factor for Later Cardiovascular Diseases: The Repeated Overshoot Theory." *International Journal of Obesity (London)* 30, suppl. 4 (December 2006): S58–66.

Montani, J. P., Y. Schutz, and Abdul G. Dulloo. "Dieting and Weight Cycling as Risk Factors for Cardiometabolic Diseases: Who is Really at Risk?" abstract. *Obesity Reviews* 16, suppl. 1 (February 2015): 7–18. http://dx.doi.org/10.1111/obr.12251.

Moore, Margaret, and Bob Tschannen-Moran. *Coaching Psychology Manual.* Philidelphia: Wolters Kluwer, 2010.

Moore, Margaret, Erika Jackson, and Bob Tschannen-Moran. *Coaching Psychology Manual.* 2nd ed. Philadelphia: Wolters Kluwer, 2016.

"NCCHWC Announces Launch of National Certification for Professional Health and Wellness Coaches." Press release of April 30, 2015. Accessed April 10, 2016. http://www.ncchwc.org/PR043015.pdf.

Neff, Kristin. "The 5 Myths of Self-Compassion: What Keeps Us from Being Kinder to Ourselves?" *Psychotherapy Networker*, September/October 2015.

Neff, Kristin. *Self-Compassion: The Proven Power of Being Kind to Yourself.* New York: William Morrow, 2011.

Neumark-Sztainer, Dianne, Melanie Wall, Jia Guo, Mary Story, Jess Haines, and Marla Eisenberg. "Obesity, Disordered Eating, and Eating Disorders in a Longitudinal Study of Adolescents: How Do Dieters Fare Five Years Later?" abstract. *Journal of the American Dietetic Association* 106, no. 4 (April 2006): 559–68. http://dx.doi.org/10.1016/j.jada.2006.01.003.

Neumark-Sztainer, Dianne, Melanie Wall, Nicole Larson, Marla Eisenberg, and Katie Loth. "Dieting and Disordered Eating Behaviors from Adolescence to Young Adulthood: Findings from a 10-Year Longitudinal Study." *Journal of the American Dietetic Association* 111, no. 7 (July 2011): 1004–11. http://dx.doi.org/10.1016/j.jada.2011.04.012.

Nicol, Ginger. "Hormones and Binge Eating Disorder." Eating Disorder Hope, October 2015. Accessed October 1, 2015. http://www.eatingdisorderhope.com/information/binge-eating-disorder/bed-research-what-do-we-know/hormones-binge-eating-disorder.

"Obesity and Depression." *ConscienHealth.* Accessed September 27, 2015. http://conscienhealth.org/2015/03/obesity-and-depression-co-conspirators/.

"Obesity and Overweight." World Health Organization website. Accessed March 31, 2016. http://www.who.int/mediacentre/factsheets/fs311/en/.

"Obesity Facts." Centers for Disease Control and Prevention website. Accessed August 5, 2016. https://www.cdc.gov/healthyschools/obesity/facts.htm.

Olshansky, S. Jay, Douglas J. Passaro, Ronald C. Hershow, Jennifer Layden, Bruce A. Carnes, Jacob Brody, Leonard Hayflick, Robert N. Butler, David B. Allison, and David S. Ludwig. "A Potential Decline in Life Expectancy in the United States in the 21st Century." *New England Journal of Medicine* 352 (2005): 1138–45. http://dx.doi.org/10.1056/NEJMsr043743.

Orbach, Susie. *Fat Is a Feminist Issue: The Anti-Diet Guide for Women*, 99–122. New York: Galahad Books, 1997.

O'Rourke, Robert W., Jason Andrus, Brian S. Diggs, Mark Scholz, Donald B. McConnell, and Clifford W. Deveney. "Perioperative Morbidity Associated with Bariatric Surgery: An Academic Center Experience," abstract. *Archives of Surgery* 141, no. 3 (March 2006): 262–68. http://dx.doi.org/10.1001/archsurg.141.3.262.

Parker-Pope, Tara. The Well Column. "Are Doctors Nicer to Thinner Patients?" April 29, 2013. http://well.blogs.nytimes.com/2013/04/29/overweight-patients-face-bias/?_r=0.

Pierpont, Yvonne N., et al. "Obesity and Surgical Wound Healing: A Current Review." *ISRN Obesity* (2014): 1–13. http://dx.doi.org/10.1155/2014/638936.

Pink, Daniel H. *Drive: The Surprising Truth about What Motivates Us.* New York: Riverhead Books, 2009.

Pittman, Genevra. "Patients Often Biased against Fat Doctors, Too." Reuters, April 12, 2013. http://www.reuters.com/article/2013/04/12/us-patients-fat-doctors-idUSBRE93B0S820130412.

Polak, Rani, Rachele M. Pojednic, and Edward M. Phillips. "Lifestyle Medicine Education." *American Journal of Lifestyle Medicine* 9, no. 5 (September 2015): 361–67. doi:10.1177/1559827615580307.

Polak, Rani, Edward M. Phillips, Julia Nordgren, and David Eisenberg. "Health-Related Culinary Education: A Summary of Representative Emerging Programs for Health Professionals and Patients." *Global Advances in Health and Medicine* 5, no. 1 (January 2016): 61–68. doi:10.7453/gahmj.2015.128.

Pollak, Kathryn I., Stewart C. Alexander, Cynthia J. Coffman, James A. Tulsky, Pauline Lyna, Rowena J. Dolor, Iguehi E. James, Rebecca J. Namenek Brouwer, Justin R. E. Manusov, and Truls Østbye. "Physician Communication Techniques and Weight Loss in Adults: Project CHAT." *American Journal of Preventive Medicine* 39, no. 4 (2010): 321–28.

Prochaska, J. O., and C. C. DiClemente. "Stages and Process of Self-Change of Smoking: Toward an Integrative Model of Change." *Journal of Consulting and Clinical Psychology* 51, no. 3 (1983): 390–95.

"Progress on Obesity." Centers for Disease Control and Prevention. Accessed March 21, 2016. http://www.cdc.gov/vitalsigns/childhoodobesity/.

Prynne, Miranda. "Overweight Doctors and Nurses Told to Slim Down by NHS Chief." *Telegraph*, July 30, 2014. http://www.telegraph.co.uk/news/nhs/10999437/Overweight-doctors-and-nurses-told-to-slim-down-by-NHS-chief.html.

Puhl, Rebecca M., and Chelsea A. Heuer. "Obesity Stigma: Important Considerations for Public Health." *American Journal of Public Health* 100, no. 6 (June 2010): 1019–28. http://www.gatherthepeople.org/Downloads/OBESITY_STIGMA.pdf.

Puhl, Rebecca M., J. L. Peterson, and J. Luedicke. "Motivating or Stigmatizing? Public Perceptions of Weight-related Language Used by Health Providers," abstract. *International Journal of Obesity* 37 (2013): 612–19. doi:10.1038/ijo.2012.110.

Raab, Kelley. "Mindfulness, Self-Compassion, and Empathy among Health Care Professionals: A Review of the Literature." *Journal of Health Care Chaplaincy* 20, no. 3 (2014): 95–108. http://dx.doi.org/10.1080/08854726.2014.913876.

Ramzi, Amri, Liliana Bordeianou, Patricia Sylla, and David Berger. "Obesity, Outcomes and Quality of Care: Body Mass Index Increases the Risk of Wound-Related Complications in Colon Cancer Surgery," abstract. *American Journal of Surgery* 207, no. 1 (January 2014): 17–23.

Rippe, James, ed. *Lifestyle Medicine, 2nd ed.* Boca Raton: Taylor & Francis Group, CBC Press, 2013.

Rollnick, Stephen, William R. Miller, and Christopher C. Butler. *Motivational Interviewing in Health Care: Helping Patients Change Behavior.* New York: The Guilford Press, 2008.

Rosenberg, Marshall B. *Nonviolent Communication: A Language of Life.* 3rd ed. Encinitas, CA: Puddledancer Press, 2015.

Russell, Christine. "Doctors, Practice What You Preach." *Atlantic,* June 12, 2012. Accessed June 12, 2012. http://www.theatlantic.com/health/archive/2012/06/doctors-practice-what-you-preach/258379/.

Saad, Lydia. "To Lose Weight, Americans Rely More on Dieting than Exercise." *Wellbeing.* Accessed October 8, 2015. http://www.gallup.com/poll/150986/lose-weight-americans-rely-dieting-exercise.aspx.

Sabgir, David. Walk With a Doc. http://walkwithadoc.org/who-we-are/metrics/.

Sabin, Janice A., Maddalena Marini, and Brian A. Nosek. "Implicit and Explicit Anti-Fat Bias among a Large Sample of Medical Doctors by BMI, Race/Ethnicity and Gender." Edited by Richard Fielding. *PLoS One* 7, no. 11 (November 7, 2012). http://www.ncbi.nlm.nih.gov/pmc/articles/PMC3492331/.

Seger, Carol A., and Brian J. Spiering. "A Critical Review of Habit Learning and the Basil Ganglia." *Frontiers in Systems Neuroscience* 4, no. 66 (2011): 1–9. Accessed March 30, 2016. http://dx.doi.org/10.3389/fnsys.2011.00066.

Seppala, Emma M., Cendri A. Hutcherson, Dong T. H. Nguyen, James R. Doty, and James J. Gross. "Loving-kindness Meditation: A Tool to Improve Healthcare Provider Compassion, Resilience, and Patient Care." *Journal of Compassionate Health Care* 1 (2014): 5. doi:10.1186/s40639-014-0005-9.

Shute, Nancy. "Fat Doctors Make Fat Patients Feel Better, and Worse." NPR, June 5, 2013. http://www.npr.org/sections/health-shots/2013/06/05/188920874/fat-doctors-make-fat-patients-feel-better-and-worse.

Staycer, Nancy. "Co-occurring Borderline Personality Disorder and Eating Disorders." Eating Disorder Hope. Accessed November 28, 2015. http://www.eatingdisorderhope.com/treatment-for-eating-disorders/co-occurring-dual-diagnosis/trauma-ptsd/co-occurring-borderline-personality-disorder-and-eating-disorders.

Sumithran Priya, and Joseph Proietto. "The Defence of Body Weight: A Physiological Basis for Weight Re-Gain after Weight Loss." *Clinical Science* 124, no. 4 (February 2013): 231–41.

Sumithran, Priya, Luke A. Prendergast, Elizabeth Delbridge, Katrina Purcell, Arthur Shulkes, Adamandia Kriketos, and Joseph Proietto. "Long-Term Persistence of Hormonal Adaptations to Weight Loss." *New England Journal of Medicine* 365, no. 17 (October 27, 2011): 1597–604. http://dx.doi.org/10.1056/NEJMoa1105816.

"Symptoms of Borderline Personality Disorder." Silver Hill Hospital. Accessed October 2, 2015. https://www.silverhillhospital.org/about-silver-hill/blog/july-2015-(1)/what-is-borderline-personality-disorder.

Taitz, Jennifer. *End Emotional Eating: Using Dialectical Behavioral Therapy Skills to Cope with Difficult Emotions and Develop a Healthy Relationship to Food.* Oakland: New Harbinger Publications, 2012.

Teachman, B. A., and K. D. Brownell. "Implicit Anti-Fat Bias among Health Professionals: Is Anyone Immune?" *International Journal of Obesity* 25, no. 10 (October 2001). http://psycnet.apa.org/psycinfo/2009-02133-002.

Teixeira, Pedro J., Eliana Carraça, Marta M. Marques, Harry Rutter, Jean-Michel Oppert, Ilse De Bourdeaudhuij, Jeroen Lakerveld, and Johannes Brug. "Successful Behavior Change in Obesity Interventions in Adults: A Systematic Review of Self-Regulation Mediators." *BMC Medicine* 13, no. 84 (April 2015). http://dx.doi.org/10.1186/s12916-015-0323-6.

Thomas, E. Louise, Gary Frost, Simon D. Tayor-Robinson, and Jimmy D. Bell. "The Missing Risk: MRI and MRS Phenotyping of Abdominal Adiposity and Ectopic Fat." *Obesity* 20 (2012): 76–87.

Tomiyama, A. Janet, Traci Mann, Danielle Vinas, Jeffrey M. Hunger, Jill DeJager, and Shelley E. Taylor. "Low Calorie Dieting Increases Cortisol." *Psychosomatic Medicine* 72, no. 4 (May 2010): 357–64. http://dx.doi.org/10.1097/PSY.0b013e3181d9523c.

Tracy, Brian. *Change Your Thinking, Change Your Life: How to Unlock Your Full Potential for Success and Achievement.* New York: MJF Books, 2003.

Tracy, Brian. *Goals: How to Get Everything You Want—Faster Than You Ever Thought Possible.* 2nd ed. Oakland: Berrett-Koehler Publishers, 2010.

"Trauma and Eating Disorders." National Eating Disorders Association. Accessed September 19, 2015. https://www.nationaleatingdisorders.org/sites/default/files/ResourceHandouts/TraumaandEatingDisorders.pdf.

"Trauma & PTSD Signs, Symptoms, Effects & Risk Factors." Timberline Knolls. Accessed September 20, 2015. http://www.timberlineknolls.com/trauma/signs-effects/.

Tribole, Evelyn. "Warning: Dieting Increases Your Risk of Gaining More Weight (An Update)," 2012. Retrieved November 6, 2015. https://www.intuitiveeating.com/content/warning-dieting-increases-your-risk-gaining-more-weight-update.

Tribole, Evelyn, and Elyse Resch. *Intuitive Eating: A Revolutionary Program that Works.* 3rd ed. New York: St. Martin's Griffin, 2012.

Trossman, Susan. "An Issue of Weight: Calling All Nurses to Get Healthy and Reverse a Trend." American Nurse, March 1, 2013. Accessed March 24, 2016. http://www.theamericannurse.org/index.php/2013/03/01/an-issue-of-weight/.

Tylka, Tracy L., and Ashley M. Kroon Van Diest. "The Intuitive Eating Scale–2: Item Refinement and Psychometric Evaluation with College Women and Men." *Journal of Counseling Psychology* 60, no. 1 (January 2013): 137–53. http://dx.doi.org/10.1037/a0030893. Accessed April 3, 2016. http://www.ncbi.nlm.nih.gov/pubmed/23356469.

Tylka, Tracy L., and Nichole Wood-Barcalow. "The Body Appreciation Scale-2: Item Refinement and Psychometric Evaluation." *Body Image* 12 (January 2015): 53–67. http://www.sciencedirect.com/science/article/pii/S1740144514001314.

Tylka, Tracy L., and Nichole Wood-Barcalow. "What is and What is not Positive Body Image? Conceptual Foundations and Construct Definition," *Body Image* (2015): 1–12. http://dx.doi.org/10.1016/j.bodyim.2015.04.001.

Tylka, Tracy L., Rachel A. Annunziato, Deb Burgard, Sigrún Daníelsdóttir, Ellen Shuman, Chad Davis, and Rachel M. Calogero. "The Weight-Inclusive versus Weight-Normative Approach to Health: Evaluating the Evidence for Prioritizing Well-Being over Weight Loss." *Journal of Obesity* (2014): 1–18. http://dx.doi.org/10.1155/2014/983495.

Uchino, Bert N. "Social Support and Health: A Review of Physiological Processes Potentially Underlying Links to Disease Outcomes." *Journal of Behavioral Medicine* 29, no. 4 (2006): 377–87. http://dx.doi.org/10.1007/s10865-006-9056-5.

Van Dyke, Nina, and Eric J. Drinkwater. "Relationships Between Intuitive Eating and Health Indicators: Literature Review." *Public Health Nutrition* 17, no. 8 (2013): 1757–66.

Waitley, Dennis. *The Psychology of Winning: Ten Qualities of a Total Winner.* New York: Berkeley Books, 1984.

Waller, Glenn, Emma Corstorphine, and Victoria Mountford. "The Role of Emotional Abuse in the Eating Disorders: Implications for Treatment." *Eating Disorders: The Journal of Treatment and Prevention* 15, no. 4 (2007). Accessed September 27, 2015. http://www.tandfonline.com/doi/abs/10.1080/10640260701454337?src=recsys.

Walsh, B. T., D. E. Wilfley, and J. I. Hudson. *Binge Eating Disorder: Progress in Understanding and Treatment.* West Wayne, NJ: Health Learning Systems, 2003.

Weineland, Sandra, Dag Arvidsson, Thanos P. Kakoulidis, and Joanne Dahl. "Acceptance and Commitment Therapy for Bariatric Surgery Patients, a Pilot RCT." *Obesity Research & Clinical Practice* 6, no. 1 (January–March 2012): e1–90. http://dx.doi.org10.1016/j.orcp.2011.04.004.

Weir, Kirstein. "Feel Like a Fraud." *American Psychological Association*, November 2013. Accessed October 8, 2015. http://www.apa.org/gradpsych/2013/11/fraud.aspx.

"What is CBT?" Beck Institute. Accessed September 15, 2015. http://www.beckinstitute.org/history-of-cbt/.

"What is Wellness Coaching?" Real Balance. Accessed March 29, 2016. https://www.realbalance.com/what-is-wellness-coaching.

"Why is Lifestyle Medicine Essential to Sustainable Health and Health Care?" American College of Lifestyle Medicine. Accessed March 1, 2016. http://www.lifestylemedicine.org/What-is-Lifestyle-Medicine.

Williams, Geoff. "The Heavy Price of Losing Weight." *U.S. News and World Report*, January 2, 2013. Accessed November 5, 2015. http://money.usnews.com/money/personal-finance/articles/2013/01/02/the-heavy-price-of-losing-weight.

Wolpert, Stuart. "Dieting Does Not Work, UCLA Researchers Report." UCLA Newsroom, April 3, 2007. Accessed October 29, 2015. http://newsroom.ucla.edu/releases/Dieting-Does-Not-Work-UCLA-Researchers-7832.

Wylie, Mary Sykes. "Can Childhood Trauma Lead to Adult Obesity? How One Study Exposed the Connection Between Early Life Abuse and Weight Gain." Psychotherapy Networker, September 24, 2015. Accessed September 30, 2015. https://www.psychotherapynetworker.org/blog/details/641/can-childhood-trauma-lead-to-adult-obesity.

Zhu, D. Q., I. J. Norman, and A. E. White. "The Relationship Between Doctors' and Nurses' Own Weight Status and Their Weight Management Practices: A Systematic Review." *Obesity Reviews*, March 2, 2011. Accessed October 27, 2015. http://onlinelibrary.wiley.com/doi/10.1111/j.1467-789X.2010.00821.x/abstract.

# Resource List

## BOOKS

*Appetites—On the Search for True Nourishment* by Geneen Roth, Plume, New York, 1996.

*BodyLove—Learning to Like Our Looks and Ourselves—A Practical Guide for Women* by Rita Freedman, Harper & Row, New York, 1988.

*Body of Truth: How Science, History and Culture Drive Our Obsession with Weight and What We Can Do about It* by Harriet Brown, Da Capo Lifelong Books, Boston, MA, 2015.

*Body Respect—What Conventional Health Books Get Wrong, Leave Out, and Just Plain Fail to Understand about Weight* by Linda Bacon and Lucy Aphramor, BenBella Book, Texas, 2014.

*Breaking Free from Compulsive Eating* by Geneen Roth, Bobbs-Merrill Co., New York, 1984.

*Change Your Thinking, Change Your Life: How to Unlock Your Full Potential for Success and Achievement* by Brian Tracy, MJF Books, New York, 2003.

*Coaching Psychology Manual* by Margaret Moore and Bob Tschannen-Moran, Wolters Kluwer, Philadelphia, 2010.

*Coaching Psychology Manual*, 2nd ed., by Margaret Moore, Erika Jackson, and Bob Tschannen-Moran, Wolters Kluwer, Philadelphia, 2016.

*Eat What You Love, Love What You Eat* by Michelle May, GreenLeaf Book Group Press, Austin, 2010.

*Eating Mindfully—How to End Mindless Eating and Enjoy a Balanced Relationship with Food* by Susan Albers, New Harbinger, California, 2003.

*Embody—Learning to Love Your Unique Body (and Quiet that Critical Voice!)* by Connie Sobczak, Gürze Books, California, 2014.

*Emotional Intelligence*, 10th Anniversary edition, by Daniel Goleman, Bantam Dell, New York, 2005.

*End Emotional Eating: Using Dialectical Behavioral Therapy Skills to Cope with Difficult Emotions and Develop a Healthy Relationship to Food* by Jennifer Taitz, New Harbinger Publications, California, 2012.

*Fat Is a Feminist Issue—A Self-Help Guide for Compulsive Eaters*, edition with new introduction, by Susie Orbach, Berkley Books, New York, 1990.

*Feeding the Hungry Heart—The Experience of Compulsive Eating* by Geneen Roth, Plume, New York, 1982.

*50 Ways to Soothe Yourself without Food* by Susan Albers, New Harbinger, California, 2009.

*The Food & Feelings Workbook—A Full Course Meal on Emotional Health* by Karen R. Koenig, Gürze Books, California, 2007.

*French Toast for Breakfast—Declaring Peace with Emotional Eating*, second revised edition, by Mary Anne Cohen, New Forge Press, New York, 2016.

*Goals! How to Get Everything You Want—Faster Than You Ever Thought Possible*, second edition, by Brian Tracy, Berrett-Koehler Publishers, Oakland, 2010.

*Health at Every Size—The Surprising Truth about Your Weight* by Linda Bacon, BenBella Books, Texas, 2008.

*Intuitive Eating—A Revolutionary Program That Works* by Evelyn Tribole and Elyse Resch, St. Martin's Paperbacks, New York, 1995.

*Lasagna for Lunch—Declaring Peace with Emotional Eating* by Mary Anne Cohen, New Forge Press, New York, 2013.

*Lifestyle Medicine, 2nd ed.* by James Rippe, Taylor & Francis Group, CBC Press, Boca Raton, FL, 2013.

*Mindset: How We Can Learn to Fulfill Our Potential* by Carol S. Dweck, Ballantine Books, New York, 2007.

*Motivational Interviewing in Health Care: Helping Patients Change Behavior* by Stephen Rollnick, William R. Miller, and Christopher C. Butler, The Guilford Press, New York, 2008.

*Nice Girls Finish Fat—Put Yourself First and Change Your Eating Forever* by Karen R. Koenig, Simon & Schuster, New York, 2009.

*Nonviolent Communication: A Language of Life*, 3rd ed., by Marshall B. Rosenberg, Puddledancer Press, Encinitas, CA, 2015.

*On Eating—Change Your Eating, Change Your Life* by Susie Orbach, Penguin Books, New York, 2002.

*Outsmarting Overeating—Boost Your Life Skills, End Your Food Problems* by Karen R. Koenig, New World Library, California, 2015.

*The Rules of "Normal" Eating—A Commonsense Approach for Dieters, Overeaters, Undereaters, Emotional Eaters, and Everyone in Between* by Karen R. Koenig, Gürze Books, California, 2005.

*Rethinking Thin—The New Science of Weight Loss and the Myths and Realities of Dieting* by Gina Kolata, Picador/Farrar, Strauss & Giroux, New York, 2007.

*Secrets from the Eating Lab—The Science of Weight Loss, the Myth of Willpower, and Why You should Never Diet Again* by Traci Mann, Harper Wave/Harper Collins, New York, 2015.

*The Self-Compassion Diet—A Step-by-Step Program to Lose Weight with Loving Kindness* by Jean Fain, Sounds True, Inc., Colorado, 2011.

*Self Compassion: The Proven Power of Being Kind to Yourself* by Kristin Neff, William Morrow, New York, 2011.

*Starting Monday—Seven Keys to a Permanent, Positive Relationship with Food* by Karen R. Koenig, Gürze Books, California, 2013.

*Wellness, Not Weight—Health at Every Size and Motivational Interviewing*, edited by Ellen Glovsky, Cognella, California, 2014.

*What Every Therapist Needs to Know about Treating Eating and Weight Issues* by Karen R. Koenig, W.W. Norton Co., New York, 2008.

*When Food Is Love—Exploring the Relationship Between Eating and Intimacy* by Geneen Roth, Penguin Group, New York, 1991.

*When Women Stop Hating Their Bodies—Freeing Yourself from Food and Weight Obsession* by Jane R. Hirschmann and Carol H. Munter, Fawcett/Ballantine Publisher Group, New York, 1995.

*When You Eat at the Refrigerator, Pull Up a Chair* by Geneen Roth, Hyperion Books, New York, 1998.

*Why Weight?—A Workbook for Ending Compulsive Eating* by Geneen Roth, Plume, New York, 1989.

## WEBSITES

http://www.amihungry.com

http://www.bedaonline.com

http://www.body-wise-perfect-size.com

http://www.thecenterformindfuleating.org

http://www.davidkatzmd.com

http://www.deliberatelifewellness.com

http://www.eatingdisorderhope.com/information

http://www.eatingdisordersblogs.com

http://www.eatingmindfully.com

http://www.edcatalogue.com

http://www.edreferral.com

http://www.emotionaleating.org

http://www.feedingourselves.com

http://www.fitwoman.com

http://www.gurzebooks.com

http://www.haescommunity.org

http://www.harvardlifestylemedicine.org

http://www.hungryforsuccess.com

http://www.instituteofcoaching.org

http://www.instituteoflifestylemedicine.org

http://www.intuitiveeating.com

http://www.jeanfain.com

http://www.karenrkoenig.com

http://www.lifestylemedicine.org

http://www.lifestylemedicineeducation.org

http://www.motivationalinterviewing.org

http://www.nationaleatingdisorders.org

http://www.ncchwc.org

http://www.paigeomahoneymd.com

http://www.prochange.com/transtheoretical-model-of-behavior-change

http://www.secretsfromtheeatinglab.com

http://www.walkwithadoc.org

http://www.wellcoachesschool.com

http://www.u.osu.edu/tracyltylka/scales-developed

## JOURNAL ARTICLES

"National Training and Education Standards for Health and Wellness Coaching: The Path to National Certification," by Meg Jordan, Ruth Q. Wolever, Karen Lawson, and Margaret Moore, *Global Advances in Health and Medicine* 4, no. 3 (May 2015): 46–56. doi:10.7453/gahmj.2015.039.

"The Weight-Inclusive Versus Weight-Normative Approach to Health: Evaluating the Evidence for Prioritizing Well-Being Over Weight Loss," by Tracy L. Tylka, Rachel A. Annunziato, Deb Burgard, Sigrún Daníelsdóttir, Ellen Shuman, Chad Davis, and Rachel M. Calogero, *Journal of Obesity* (2014): 1–18. http://dx.doi.org/10.1155/2014/983495.

# Index

# About the Authors

**Karen R. Koenig**, M.Ed., LCSW, is a psychotherapist, blogger, educator, and international author of six previous books on eating, weight, and body image. An expert on the psychology of eating—the why and how, not the what of it— she has been working in the field of eating disorders for over thirty years. Karen has written for *Social Work Today, Social Work Focus,* and *Eating Disorders Today*, and she has been quoted in the *Boston Globe,* the *Boston Herald*, the *Ladies Home Journal*, the *Wall Street Journal, Berner Zeitung, Women's Health,* and the *Sarasota Herald-Tribune*. Her mission is to help dysregulated eaters become "normal" eaters. She practices out of Sarasota, Florida, and her website is http://www.karenrkoenig.com.

**Paige O'Mahoney**, M.D., CHWC, is a physician, health and wellness coach, certified Intuitive Eating counselor, and founder of Deliberate Life Wellness, LLC, a collaborative coaching and medical education initiative whose mission is to promote compassionate care, highlight resources and experts, and change the conversation about weight and wellness among patients, clinicians, and policy makers. Paige is a member of the American College of Lifestyle Medicine (ACLM) and the Lifestyle Medicine Education Collaborative (LMEd). In addition to her coaching practice, Paige conducts group workshops, develops curricular and continuing medical and health education

training materials, and speaks to both professional and lay audiences on topics related to healing overeating and creating a deliberate, satisfying life. Her
websites are http://www.paigeomahoneymd.com and http://www.deliber-
atelifewellness.com.